Melanoma

Edited by Ahmed Lasfar
and Karine Cohen-Solal

Published in London, United Kingdom

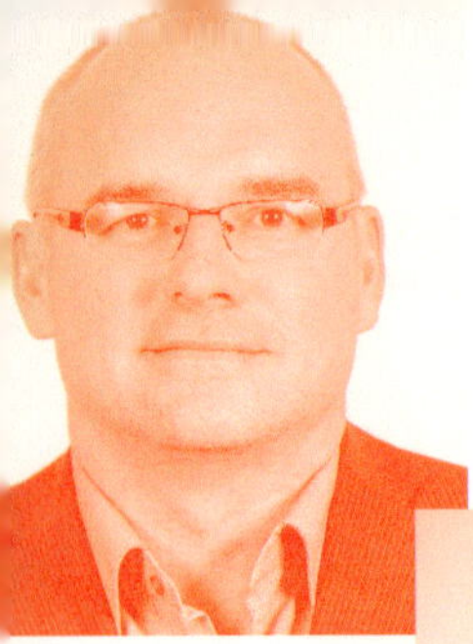
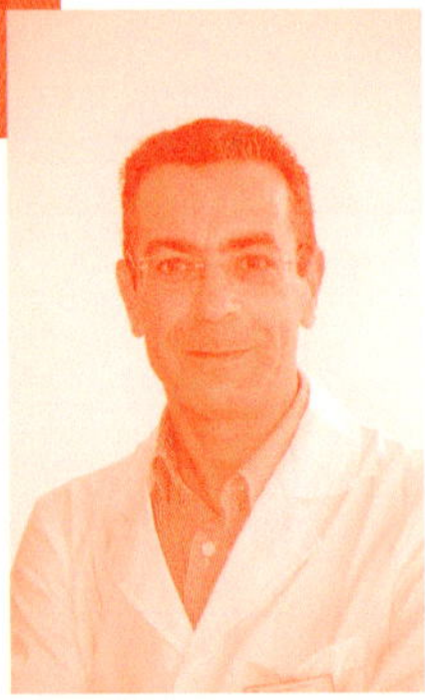
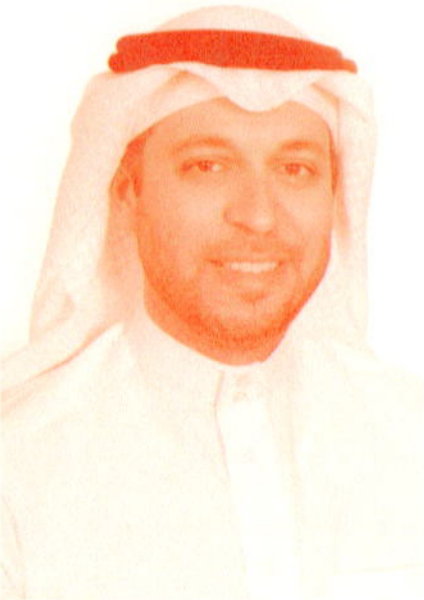
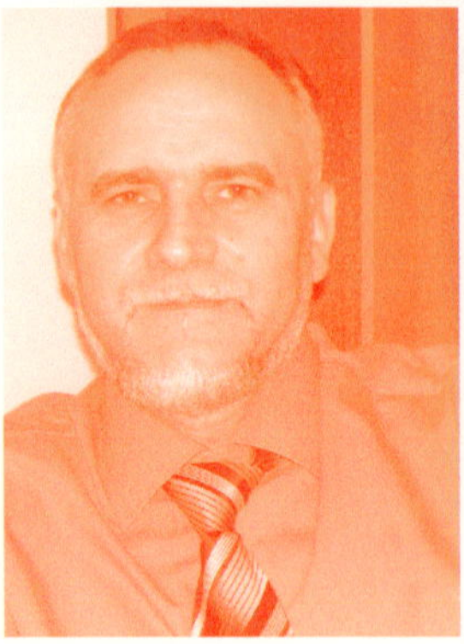
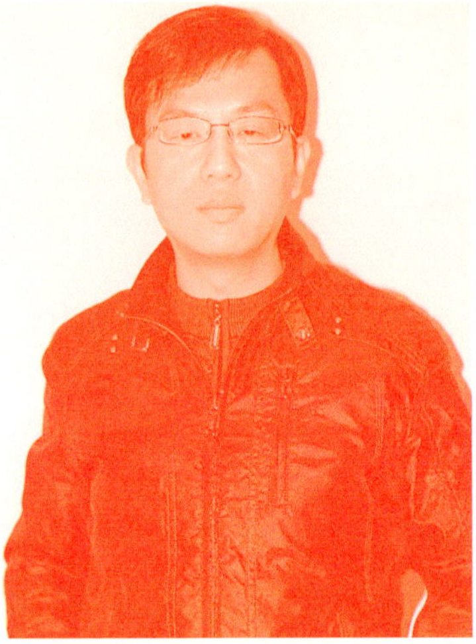
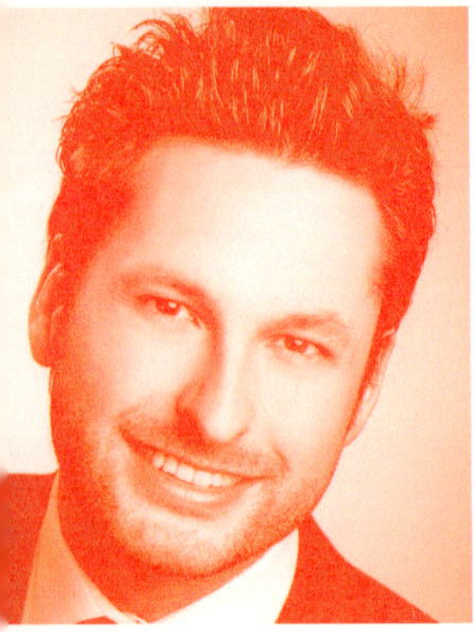
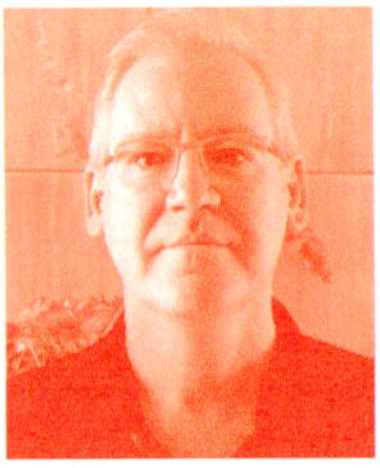

IntechOpen

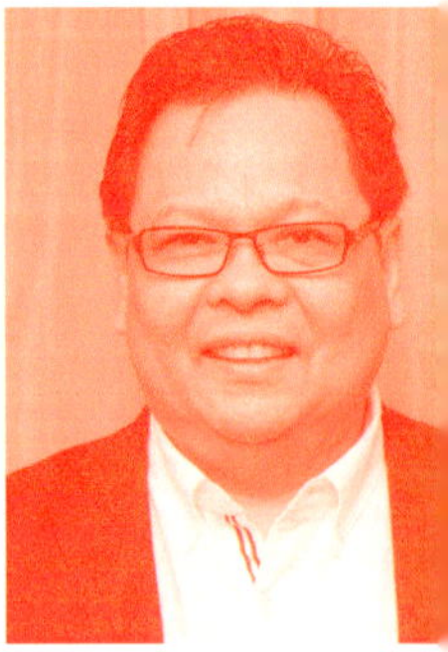
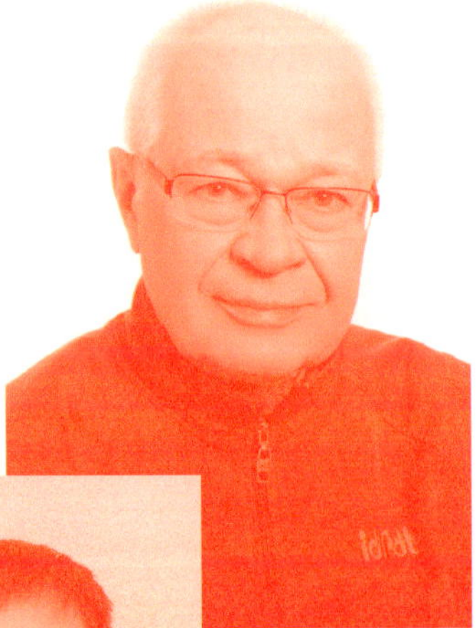
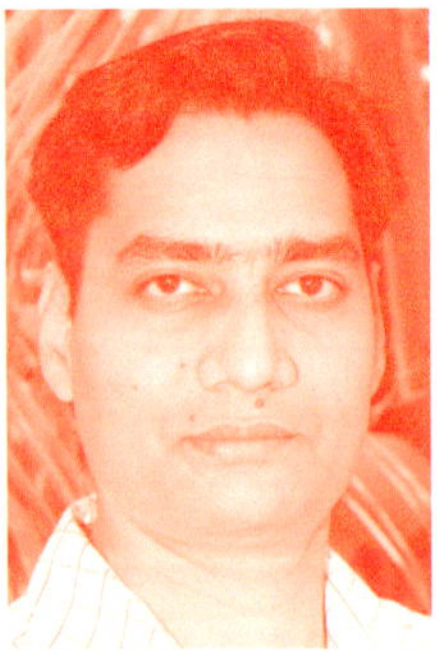
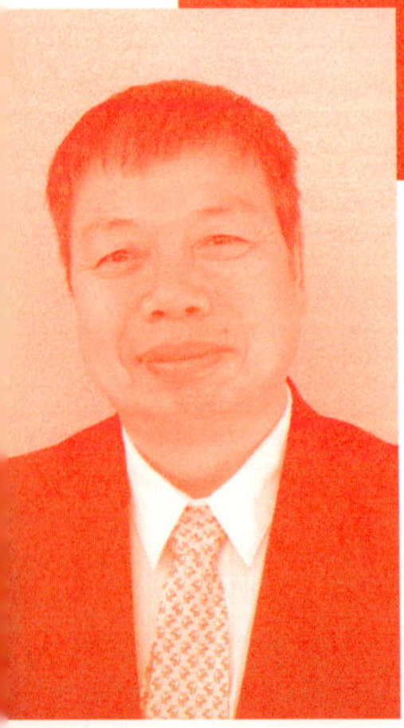
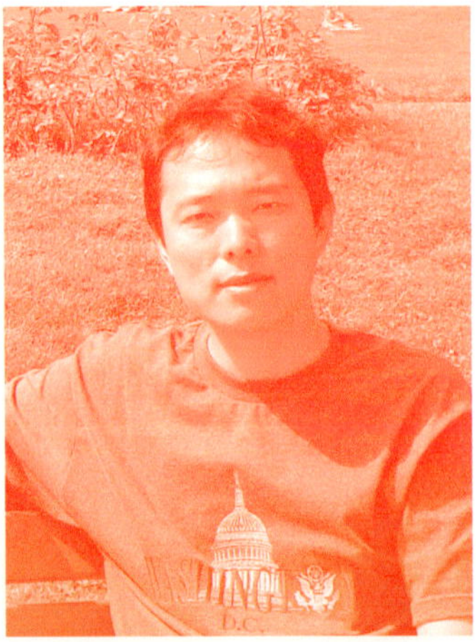
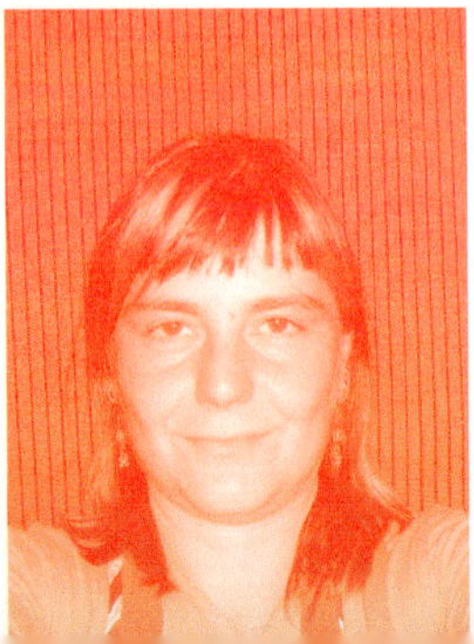

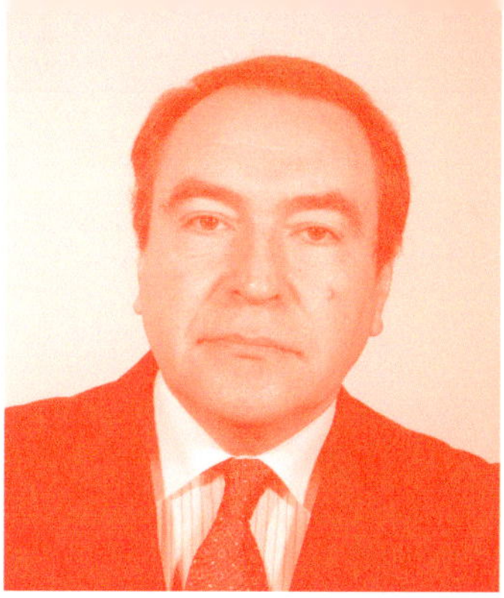
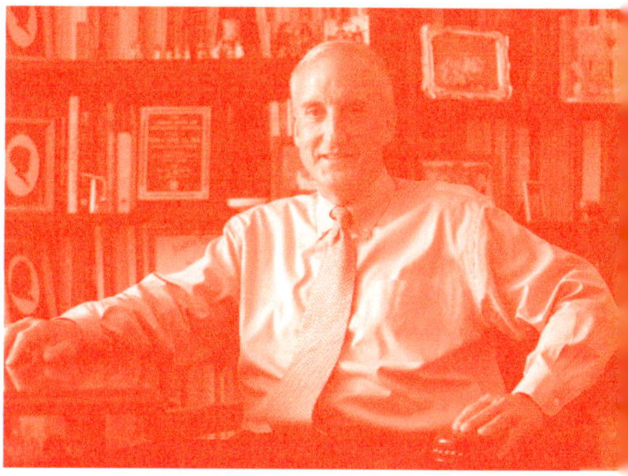
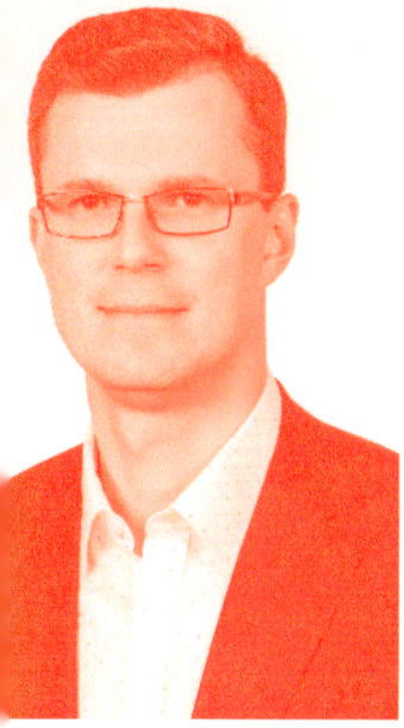
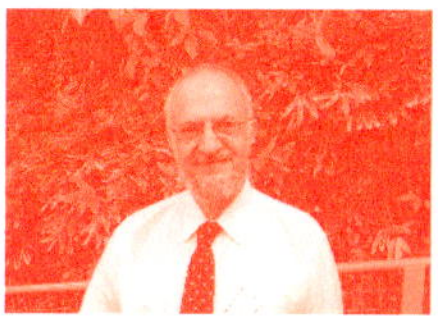
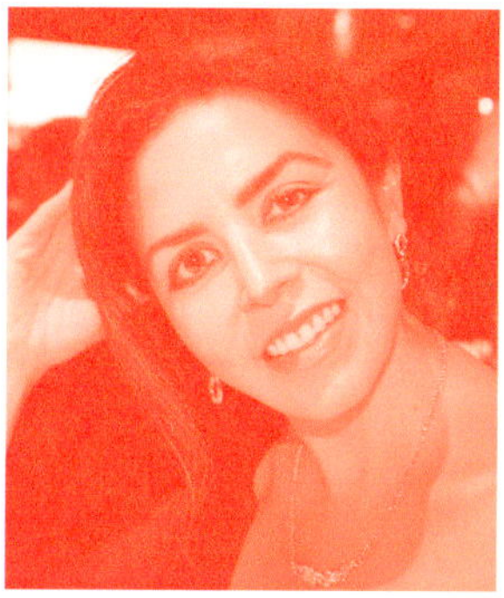

Supporting open minds since 2005

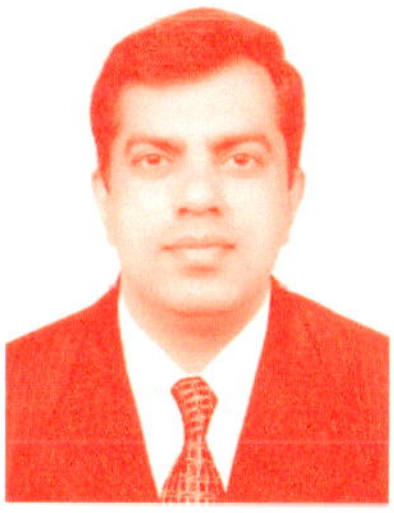
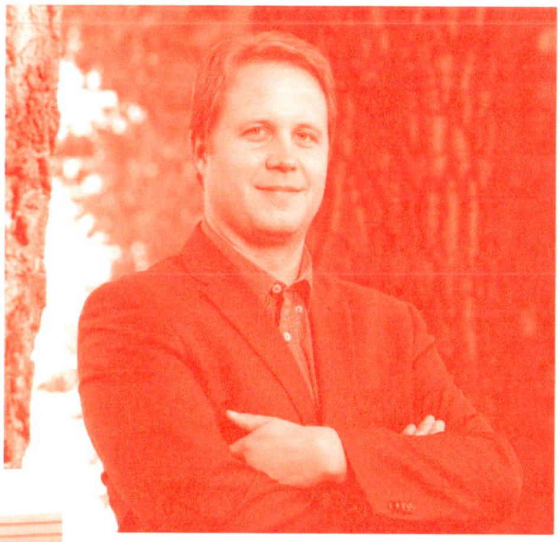
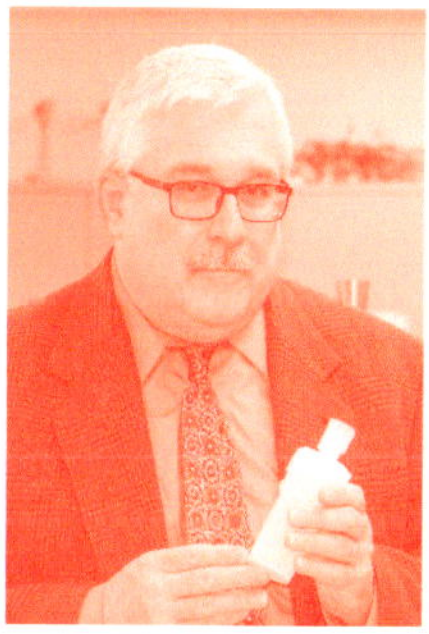
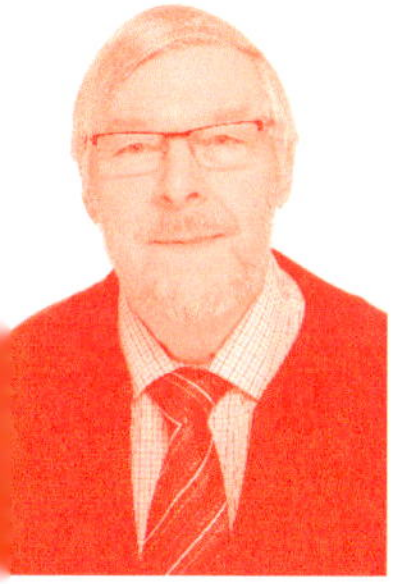
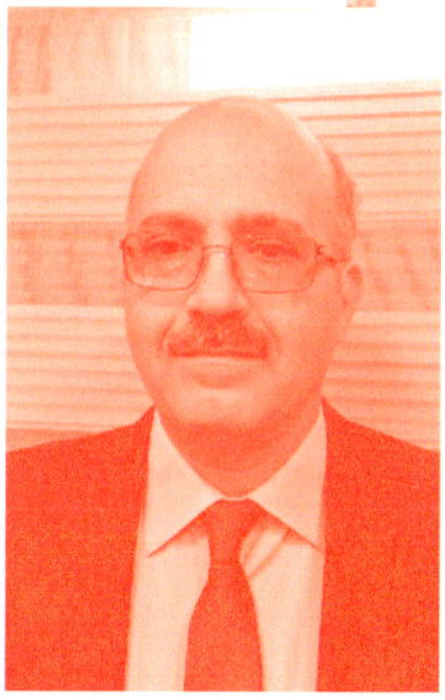
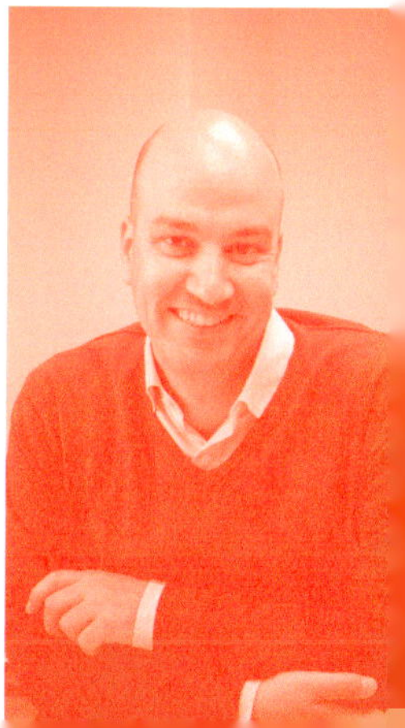
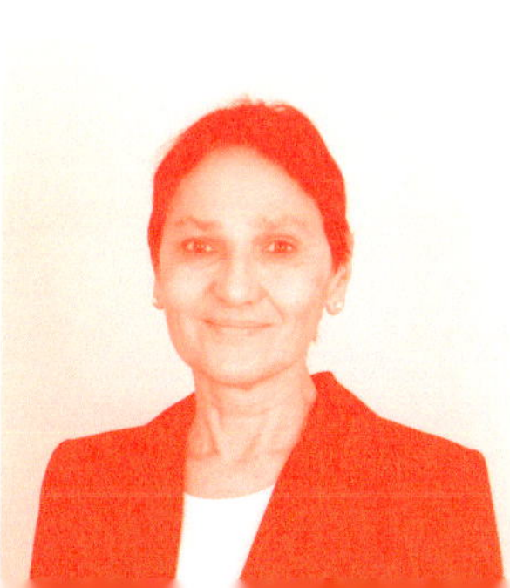

Melanoma
http://dx.doi.org/10.5772/intechopen.91524
Edited by Ahmed Lasfar and Karine Cohen-Solal

Contributors
Alena Furdova, Kristína Horkovičová, Dace Pjanova, Ninel M. Vainshelbaum, Kristine Salmina, Jekaterina Erenpreisa, Harika Regani, Santosh G. Honavar, Rahul Gupta, Nalini Bansal, Houssem Ammar, Jyoti Koli, Ullyanov Bezerra Toscano Mendonca, Julia Soffientini, Keren Cozer, Victoria Ficher Barbosa, Ahmed Lasfar, Karine Cohen Solal, Rachael Pulica

First published in London, United Kingdom, 2021 by IntechOpen
IntechOpen is the global imprint of INTECHOPEN LIMITED, registered in England and Wales, registration number: 11086078, 5 Princes Gate Court, London, SW7 2QJ, United Kingdom
Printed in Croatia

British Library Cataloguing-in-Publication Data
A catalogue record for this book is available from the British Library

Additional hard and PDF copies can be obtained from orders@intechopen.com

Melanoma
Edited by Ahmed Lasfar and Karine Cohen-Solal
p. cm.
Print ISBN 978-1-83880-878-5
Online ISBN 978-1-83880-879-2
eBook (PDF) ISBN 978-1-83880-880-8

For EU product safety concerns:
IN TECH d.o.o., Prolaz Marije Krucifikse Kozulić 3, 51000 Rijeka, Croatia, info@intechopen.com or visit our website at intechopen.com.

Meet the editors

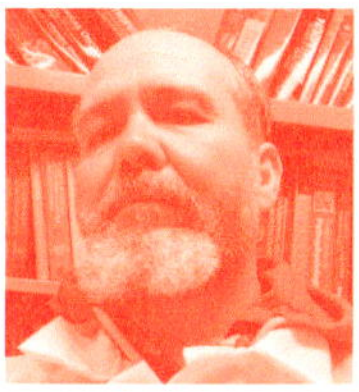

Dr. Ahmed Lasfar is a Cancer Immunologist and a leading expert on melanoma. He is a full member of the Rutgers-Cancer Institute of New Jersey, principal investigator, and a faculty member at Ernest Mario School of Pharmacy, Rutgers University, New Jersey. Dr. Lasfar's laboratory focuses on understanding the immune mechanisms controlling cancer development and metastasis. In addition to melanoma, Dr. Lasfar's laboratory is studying hepatocellular carcinoma and breast cancer. Dr. Lasfar has edited several books and research topics in cancer. He is an editor, board member, and reviewer of relevant international journals and foundations. Dr. Lasfar also serves as a consultant scientific adviser for the pharmaceutical industry. Dr. Lasfar obtained his undergraduate and graduate degrees in France from Paris Rene Descartes University and Denis Diderot University. He completed his postdoctoral training in cancer immunology at Robert Wood Johnson Medical School in New Jersey.

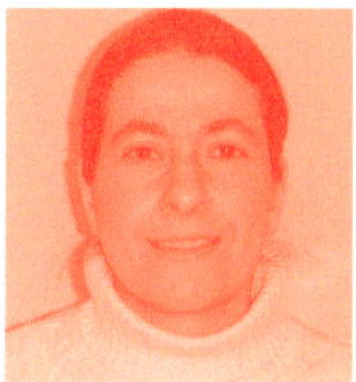

Dr. Karine Cohen-Solal is an oncologist with leading expertise in melanoma, having directed a laboratory focused on melanoma research and cell signaling. Currently, she is Director of Medical Strategy, Oncology, at Physicians' Education Resource, New Jersey, and adjunct faculty in the Department of Pharmacology and Toxicology, Rutgers, The State University of New Jersey. Dr. Cohen-Solal graduated from Paris University, France, and completed her postdoctoral training at Ernest Mario School of Pharmacy, Rutgers. Dr. Cohen-Solal received several awards including a Research Scholar Grant from the American Cancer Society and awards from the New Jersey Commission on Cancer Research and the Melanoma Research Foundation. Dr. Cohen-Solal's breakthroughs involve the identification of a new type of receptor in the genesis of melanoma, the disruption of natural tumor suppressive mechanisms in melanoma development and progression, as well as the role of oncogenic signaling in immune escape mechanisms.

Contents

Preface

Malignant melanoma is the most aggressive skin cancer. Despite this, significant progress has been achieved for patients with unresectable or advanced melanoma. The introduction of targeted therapy and, most recently, immune checkpoint blockades have revolutionized melanoma treatment, increasing patient rates of survival even in advanced disease. However, many melanoma patients are not benefiting from current therapies. The major obstacle to therapeutic success is drug resistance. The mechanisms of therapeutic resistance are under intense investigation and novel therapeutic strategies based on combining targeted therapy and immunotherapy are emerging. Many clinical trials of the combination of BRAF inhibitors and immune checkpoint inhibitors are very promising. We believe there is a brighter future for therapeutic options for malignant melanoma.

This book explores the advances and challenges associated with melanoma, including its diagnosis and management, and proposes new avenues for therapeutic opportunities, based on sustained research efforts and ever-growing technological advances.

The publication of this book was made possible by coordinated efforts and collaborations from many experts and outstanding researchers on melanoma. We thank all the contributors for their valuable studies and their wonderful efforts.

We are confident that this book provides important insights into melanoma treatment, the emergence of therapeutic resistance, and novel therapeutic strategies. We believe it will contribute to bringing answers and hope for healthcare providers, clinicians, and scientists as well as patients and their loved ones.

Dr. Ahmed Lasfar
Department of Pharmacology and Toxicology,
Ernest Mario School of Pharmacy, Rutgers,
The State University of New Jersey,
Piscataway, NJ, United States

Rutgers-Cancer Institute of New Jersey,
Rutgers University,
New Brunswick, NJ, United States

Dr. Karine Cohen Solal
Department of Pharmacology and Toxicology,
Ernest Mario School of Pharmacy, Rutgers,
The State University of New Jersey,
Piscataway, NJ, United States

Section 1

Types and Categories of Melanoma

Chapter 1

Introductory Chapter: Melanoma and Therapeutic Perspectives

Karine Cohen Solal and Ahmed Lasfar

1. Introduction

Malignant melanoma is one of the most aggressive forms of skin cancer, often leading to distal metastasis [1, 2]. Melanoma arises often from transformed melanocytes as a consequence of durable UV radiation. Unprecedented progress in the treatment of advanced melanoma occurred largely through advances in understanding how to target selective genetic mutations in patients with melanoma, and to unleash exiting anti-tumor immune responses [3–5]. While immunotherapy is characterized by induction of durable responses in a limited number of patients, targeted therapy has been characterized by high response rates [4, 5]. The introduction of targeted therapies has considerably improved survival rates in a significant proportion of patients with BRAF-mutant melanomas [6, 7]. However, drug resistance significantly weakens the efficacy of almost all current anticancer therapies [8, 9]. This resistance to therapy is generally driven by intrinsic or acquired tumor mechanisms [10]. Understand underlying mechanisms of resistance is crucial in elaborating novel therapeutic strategies (**Figure 1**).

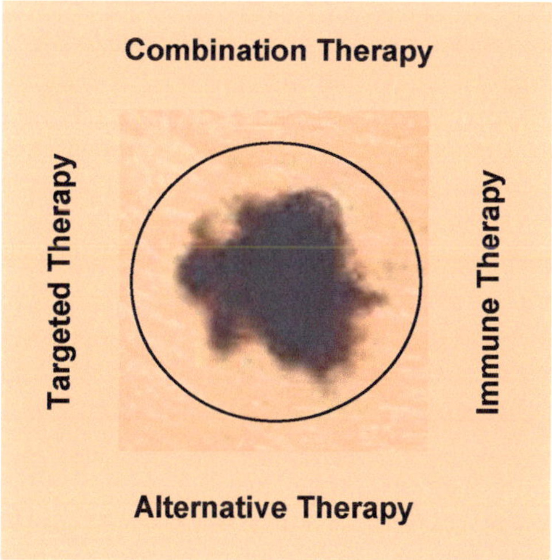

Figure 1.
Current melanoma therapies. Several therapies are currently used in clinic for the treatment of melanoma patients. Current therapies are based on targeted therapy, immune therapy and combination therapy, consisting on association of both targeted and immune therapies. In addition, alternative therapy. Is used in many cases of drug resistance.

2. Therapeutic resistance to targeted therapy

Emergence of drug resistance, usually within several months considerably limited expected survival benefits [8, 9]. The V600E activating mutation of BRAF (MAPK pathway effector) induces constitutive activation of the kinase in 45–60% of cutaneous melanomas, and inhibitors of BRAF, MEK or both have revolutionized the treatment of patients with BRAF-mutated melanoma [10, 11]. Some mechanisms of drug resistance have been being identified and strategies to circumvent therapy failure are being investigated in preclinical models and clinical studies [12].

Accumulating evidence demonstrated that in the context of acquired resistance, tumor cells will develop mechanisms that not only promote resistance to BRAF V600E targeted therapy but also increase invasiveness favorable to further dissemination and metastasis [10, 13, 14]. The molecular effectors involved in resistance to BRAF V600E targeted therapy are simultaneously playing key roles in melanoma cell motility and invasiveness [8, 10]. Numerous studies documented that resistance is often coupled to the development of an aggressive tumor phenotype, characterized by an active epithelial-to mesenchymal (EMT)-like process, increased motility and invasion [15, 16]. As a well-documented example, transcription factors and coactivators play an active role in resistance to BRAF V600E targeted therapy, through a large variety of mechanisms [17]. In addition to promoting adaptive or acquired resistance, the expression levels of some of these transcription factors promotes a state of intrinsic resistance in the context of melanoma cells harboring BRAF V600E mutations [18–20].

General mechanisms of BRAF inhibitor resistance involve up or down regulation of transcription factors, phosphorylation of transcription factors, as well as modulation of their subcellular localization [17–20]. These alterations are associated with diverse oncogenic mechanisms, such as induced expression of ERK kinases or stabilization of their phosphorylation, an increase and/or activation of specific receptor tyrosine kinases, such as EGFR, IGF-1R, AXL PDGFRβ, ERBB3, or the activation of the TGF-β signaling pathway [17, 19]. Moreover, G-protein-coupled receptors are being involved as a new protein class whose dysregulation underlies a cascade of transcriptional events resulting in resistance to BRAF inhibition. These studies altogether strongly suggest that the resistance mechanisms reestablish activation of the MAPK pathway, on which melanoma cells are highly dependent for survival, proliferation, aggressiveness and pro-metastatic behavior [17, 21]. In addition, reactivation of additional pathways, such as the PI3K/AKT pathway or GPCR-mediated cAMP/PKA/CREB pathway further operate for rewiring melanoma cells towards more aggressive characteristics in conjunction with drug resistance [21].

Simultaneous rewiring of oncogenic signaling pathways, phenotypic plasticity favoring pro-invasive behavior, actin remodeling and cytoskeletal tension, and bidirectional interplay between tumor cells and melanoma microenvironment, represent remaining challenges, for overcoming resistance to BRAF V600E inhibitors [22].

Other mechanisms of drug resistance have been identified in both melanoma patients and BRAF-animal models. Recently, it has been reported that BRAF interacts with GRP78 and removes its inhibitory impact on the three major ER stress sensors of UPR, PERK, IRE1α, and ATF6. Disconnection of GRP78 from these ER stress sensors stimulates UPR that consequently activates cytoprotective autophagy. Thus, inhibition of BRAF-induced ER stress-mediated autophagy can possibly resensitize BRAF mutant melanoma tumors to apoptosis [23].

Melanomas frequently display hyperactivity of nitric oxide synthase (NOS) and NADPH oxidase (NOX), which, respectively, produce nitric oxide ($NO^{\cdot}$) and superoxide ($O2^{\cdot-}$). The $NO^{\cdot}$ and $O2^{-}$ react instantaneously with each other to produce peroxynitrite ($ONOO^-$) which is the driver force of melanin chemiexcitation. Melanocytes, the skin cells, specialized in synthesizing melanin, a shield against sunlight's ultraviolet (UV) radiation. However, melanin chemiexcitation paradoxically demonstrates the melanomagenic properties of melanin. In a loop, the NOS activity regulates melanin synthesis, and melanin is utilized by the chemiexcitation pathway to generate carcinogenic melanin-carbonyls in an excited triplet state. These carbonyl compounds induce UV-specific DNA damage without UV [24].

It has been also reported that melanoma cells gain drug resistance to Temozolomide through a complex inflammatory mechanism, involving Inflammasome Sensor NLRP1 [25].

There is emergent indication that altered expression levels of microRNAs (miRNA)s induce drug-resistance in melanoma cells and that restoring adequate expression of miRNAs is critical in the re-establishment of therapeutic sensitivity [26].

3. Immunotherapy resistance

On the other hand, since the first immune checkpoint inhibitor (ICI) approval of an anti-CTL-A monoclonal antibody (mAb) in 2011 for unresectable/metastatic melanoma, the class continued to evolve, resulting in an always-changing standard of care for patients. Unfortunately, innate and acquired resistance to ICIs prevent a substantial number of patients with advanced melanoma to benefit from these clinical breakthroughs [27]. As the mechanisms responsible for both innate and acquired resistance to ICIs are further elucidated, therapeutic strategies to overcome these resistances are being clinically evaluated and will undoubtedly provide superior therapeutic efficacy [28].

As an example, clinical trials are currently evaluating inhibitors of myeloid-derived suppressors cells, which have emerged as important components in resistance to cancer immunotherapy [29, 30]. In addition, intra-tumor injection of interleukin-12, GMCSF, and Toll-like receptors (TLR9) agonists, among other agents are currently evaluated in patients with melanoma refractory to anti-PD1 blockade [31, 32]. Another approach clinically tested in patients with BRAFV600E is the triple combination of an approved anti-PD-L1 monoclonal antibody and an approved combination of BRAF inhibitor/MEK inhibitor; this triplet regimen is based on the rationale that BRAF inhibition increases the penetration of T cells into the tumors, a major factor in the ability to respond to ICIs [33]. Altogether, the different approaches aim at transforming a cold tumor, characterized by a lack or paucity of tumor T cell infiltration, into a hot, inflamed tumor.

4. Alternative therapeutic strategies

Other alternative approaches have been elaborated in the treatment of metastatic melanoma such as Photodynamic therapy (PDT), which relies on a light-activated compound to produce death-inducing amounts of reactive oxygen species (ROS) [34].

Histone Deacetylase Inhibitors have been also developed to overcome resistance to targeted and immunotherapy in Metastatic Melanoma [35].

Nanotechnology, based therapy or neoadjuvant therapy represent an active area of investigation as demonstrated by several clinical trials [36]. These novel strategies may offer a multitude of benefits which could improve the survival outcomes of melanoma patients, with low adverse effects. Their combination with immunotherapies and vaccines are expected to overcome drug resistance, offering survival benefits to a greater population of patients with advanced melanoma, while maintaining a satisfying quality of life.

5. Conclusion

The future of patients with unresectable and advanced melanoma is looking brighter than a decade ago. Besides immunotherapy revolution, promising approaches are emerging. Currently combination therapy, based on targeted therapy and immune checkpoint inhibitors is commonly recommended for increasing treatment efficacy. However, many challenges remain, regarding the mechanisms of tumorigenesis, the impact of tumor microenvironment on the immunogenicity of melanoma.

Author details

Karine Cohen Solal[1] and Ahmed Lasfar[1,2*]

1 Department of Pharmacology and Toxicology, Ernest Mario School of Pharmacy, Rutgers, The State University of New Jersey, Piscataway, NJ, United States

2 Rutgers-Cancer Institute of New Jersey, Rutgers University, New Brunswick, NJ, United States

*Address all correspondence to: lasfarah@gmail.com

References

[1] Siegel RL, Miller KD and Jemal A: Cancer statistics, 2018. CA Cancer J Clin. 68:7-30.

[2] Leonardi GC, Falzone L, Salemi R, Zanghì A, Spandidos DA, McCubrey JA, Candido S and Libra M: Cutaneous melanoma: From pathogenesis to therapy (Review). Int J Oncol. 52:1071-1080. 2018.

[3] Jenkins RW, Fisher DE. Treatment of Advanced Melanoma in 2020 and Beyond. J Invest Dermatol. 2021 Jan;141(1):23-31. doi: 10.1016/j.jid.2020.03.943. Epub 2020 Apr 5. PMID: 32268150; PMCID: PMC7541692.

[4] Massimo Ralli, Andrea Botticelli, Irene Claudia Visconti, Diletta Angeletti, Marco Fiore, Paolo Marchetti, Alessandro Lambiase, Marco de Vincentiis, Antonio Greco, "Immunotherapy in the Treatment of Metastatic Melanoma: Current Knowledge and Future Directions", Journal of Immunology Research, vol. 2020, Article ID 9235638, 12 pages, 2020.

[5] Leonardi GC, Candido S, Falzone L, Spandidos DA, Libra M. Cutaneous melanoma and the immunotherapy revolution (Review). Int J Oncol. 2020 Sep;57(3):609-618. doi: 10.3892/ijo.2020.5088. Epub 2020 Jun 25. PMID: 32582963; PMCID: PMC7384846.

[6] Falcone I, Conciatori F, Bazzichetto C, Ferretti G, Cognetti F, Ciuffreda L, Milella M. Tumor Microenvironment: Implications in Melanoma Resistance to Targeted Therapy and Immunotherapy. Cancers (Basel). 2020 Oct 6;12(10):2870. doi: 10.3390/cancers12102870. PMID: 33036192; PMCID: PMC7601592.

[7] Liguoro D, Fattore L, Mancini R, Ciliberto G. Drug tolerance to target therapy in melanoma revealed at single cell level: What next? Biochim Biophys Acta Rev Cancer. 2020 Dec;1874(2): 188440. doi: 10.1016/j.bbcan.2020.188440. Epub 2020 Sep 29. PMID: 33007433.

[8] Tangella LP, Clark ME, Gray ES. Resistance mechanisms to targeted therapy in BRAF-mutant melanoma - A mini review. Biochim Biophys Acta Gen Subj. 2021 Jan;1865(1):129736. doi: 10.1016/j.bbagen.2020.129736. Epub 2020 Sep 18. PMID: 32956754.

[9] Mazurkiewicz J, Simiczyjew A, Dratkiewicz E, Ziętek M, Matkowski R, Nowak D. Stromal Cells Present in the Melanoma Niche Affect Tumor Invasiveness and Its Resistance to Therapy. Int J Mol Sci. 2021 Jan 7;22(2):529. doi: 10.3390/ijms22020529. PMID: 33430277; PMCID: PMC7825728.

[10] Kakadia S, Yarlagadda N, Awad R, Kundranda M, Niu J, Naraev B, Mina L, Dragovich T, Gimbel M, Mahmoud F. Mechanisms of resistance to BRAF and MEK inhibitors and clinical update of US Food and Drug Administration-approved targeted therapy in advanced melanoma. Onco Targets Ther. 2018 Oct 17;11:7095-7107. doi: 10.2147/OTT.S182721. PMID: 30410366; PMCID: PMC6200076.

[11] Alqathama A. BRAF in malignant melanoma progression and metastasis: potentials and challenges. Am J Cancer Res. 2020 Apr 1;10(4):1103-1114. PMID: 32368388; PMCID: PMC7191094.

[12] Tanda ET, Vanni I, Boutros A, Andreotti V, Bruno W, Ghiorzo P, Spagnolo F. Current State of Target Treatment in BRAF Mutated Melanoma. Front Mol Biosci. 2020 Jul 14;7:154. doi: 10.3389/fmolb.2020.00154. PMID: 32760738; PMCID: PMC7371970.

[13] Ray A, Kunhiraman H, Perera RJ. The Paradoxical Behavior of

microRNA-211 in Melanomas and Other Human Cancers. Front Oncol. 2021 Feb 8;10:628367. doi: 10.3389/fonc.2020.628367. PMID: 33628737; PMCID: PMC7897698.

[14] Patton EE, Mueller KL, Adams DJ, Anandasabapathy N, Aplin AE, Bertolotto C, Bosenberg M, Ceol CJ, Burd CE, Chi P, Herlyn M, Holmen SL, Karreth FA, Kaufman CK, Khan S, Kobold S, Leucci E, Levy C, Lombard DB, Lund AW, Marie KL, Marine JC, Marais R, McMahon M, Robles-Espinoza CD, Ronai ZA, Samuels Y, Soengas MS, Villanueva J, Weeraratna AT, White RM, Yeh I, Zhu J, Zon LI, Hurlbert MS, Merlino G. Melanoma models for the next generation of therapies. Cancer Cell. 2021 Feb 4:S1535-6108(21)00055-6. doi: 10.1016/j.ccell.2021.01.011. Epub ahead of print. PMID: 33545064.

[15] Tang Y, Durand S, Dalle S, Caramel J. EMT-Inducing Transcription Factors, Drivers of Melanoma Phenotype Switching, and Resistance to Treatment. Cancers (Basel). 2020 Aug 4;12(8):2154. doi: 10.3390/cancers12082154. PMID: 32759677; PMCID: PMC7465730.

[16] Hodorogea A, Calinescu A, Antohe M, Balaban M, Nedelcu RI, Turcu G, Ion DA, Badarau IA, Popescu CM, Popescu R, Popp C, Cioplea M, Nichita L, Hulea I, Brinzea A. Epithelial-Mesenchymal Transition in Skin Cancers: A Review. Anal Cell Pathol (Amst). 2019 Dec 16;2019:3851576. doi: 10.1155/2019/3851576. PMID: 31934531; PMCID: PMC6942705.

[17] Cohen-Solal KA, Kaufman HL, Lasfar A. Transcription factors as critical players in melanoma invasiveness, drug resistance, and opportunities for therapeutic drug development. Pigment Cell Melanoma Res. 2018 Mar;31(2):241-252. doi: 10.1111/pcmr.12666. Epub 2017 Nov 15. PMID: 29090514.

[18] Hüser L, Kokkaleniou MM, Granados K, Dworacek J, Federico A, Vierthaler M, Novak D, Arkhypov I, Hielscher T, Umansky V, Altevogt P, Utikal J. HER3-Receptor-Mediated STAT3 Activation Plays a Central Role in Adaptive Resistance toward Vemurafenib in Melanoma. Cancers (Basel). 2020 Dec 14;12(12):3761. doi: 10.3390/cancers12123761. PMID: 33327495; PMCID: PMC7764938.

[19] Azimi A, Tuominen R, Costa Svedman F, Caramuta S, Pernemalm M, Frostvik Stolt M, Kanter L, Kharaziha P, Lehtiö J, Hertzman Johansson C, Höiom V, Hansson J, Egyhazi Brage S. Silencing FLI or targeting CD13/ANPEP lead to dephosphorylation of EPHA2, a mediator of BRAF inhibitor resistance, and induce growth arrest or apoptosis in melanoma cells. Cell Death Dis. 2017 Aug 31;8(8):e3029. doi: 10.1038/cddis.2017.406. PMID: 29048432; PMCID: PMC5596587.

[20] Liu L, Yue Q, Ma J, Liu Y, Zhao T, Guo W, Zhu G, Guo S, Wang S, Gao T, Li C, Shi Q. POU4F1 promotes the resistance of melanoma to BRAF inhibitors through MEK/ERK pathway activation and MITF up-regulation. Cell Death Dis. 2020 Jun 12;11(6):451. doi: 10.1038/s41419-020-2662-2. PMID: 32532957; PMCID: PMC7293281.

[21] Eddy K, Shah R, Chen S. Decoding Melanoma Development and Progression: Identification of Therapeutic Vulnerabilities. Front Oncol. 2021 Feb 4;10:626129. doi: 10.3389/fonc.2020.626129. PMID: 33614507; PMCID: PMC7891057.

[22] Dumaz N, Lebbé C. New perspectives on targeting RAF, MEK and ERK in melanoma. Curr Opin Oncol. 2021 Mar 1;33(2):120-126. doi: 10.1097/CCO.0000000000000708. PMID: 33332926.

[23] Rather RA, Bhagat M, Singh SK. Oncogenic BRAF, endoplasmic reticulum stress, and autophagy: Crosstalk and therapeutic targets in cutaneous melanoma. Mutat Res. 2020 Jul-Sep;785:108321. doi: 10.1016/j.mrrev.2020.108321. Epub 2020 Jul 7. PMID: 32800272).

[24] Premi S. Role of Melanin Chemiexcitation in Melanoma Progression and Drug Resistance. Front Oncol. 2020 Aug 6;10:1305. doi: 10.3389/fonc.2020.01305. PMID: 32850409; PMCID: PMC7425655.

[25] Zhai Z, Samson JM, Yamauchi T, Vaddi PK, Matsumoto Y, Dinarello CA, Ravindran Menon D, Fujita M. Inflammasome Sensor NLRP1 Confers Acquired Drug Resistance to Temozolomide in Human Melanoma. Cancers (Basel). 2020 Sep 4;12(9):2518. doi: 10.3390/cancers12092518. PMID: 32899791; PMCID: PMC7563249.

[26] Motti ML, Minopoli M, Di Carluccio G, Ascierto PA, Carriero MV. MicroRNAs as Key Players in Melanoma Cell Resistance to MAPK and Immune Checkpoint Inhibitors. Int J Mol Sci. 2020 Jun 26;21(12):4544. doi: 10.3390/ijms21124544. PMID: 32604720; PMCID: PMC7352536.

[27] Bagchi S, Yuan R, Engleman EG. Immune Checkpoint Inhibitors for the Treatment of Cancer: Clinical Impact and Mechanisms of Response and Resistance. Annu Rev Pathol. 2021 Jan 24;16:223-249. doi: 10.1146/annurev-pathol-042020-042741. Epub 2020 Nov 16. PMID: 33197221.

[28] Bai X, Flaherty KT. Targeted and immunotherapies in BRAF mutant melanoma: where we stand and what to expect. Br J Dermatol. 2020 Jul 11. doi: 10.1111/bjd.19394. Epub ahead of print. PMID: 32652567.

[29] Chevolet I, Speeckaert R, Schreuer M, Neyns B, Krysko O, Bachert C, Van Gele M, van Geel N, Brochez L. Clinical significance of plasmacytoid dendritic cells and myeloid-derived suppressor cells in melanoma. J Transl Med. 2015 Jan 16;13:9. doi: 10.1186/s12967-014-0376-x. PMID: 25592374; PMCID: PMC4326397.

[30] Groth C, Arpinati L, Shaul ME, Winkler N, Diester K, Gengenbacher N, Weber R, Arkhypov I, Lasser S, Petrova V, Augustin HG, Altevogt P, Utikal J, Fridlender ZG, Umansky V. Blocking Migration of Polymor phonuclear Myeloid-Derived Suppressor Cells Inhibits Mouse Melanoma Progression. Cancers (Basel). 2021 Feb 10;13(4):726. doi: 10.3390/cancers13040726. PMID: 33578808.

[31] Kim KJ, Moon D, Kong SJ, Lee YS, Yoo Y, Kim S, Kim C, Chon HJ, Kim JH, Choi KJ. Antitumor effects of IL-12 and GM-CSF co-expressed in an engineered oncolytic HSV-1. Gene Ther. 2020 Nov 4. doi: 10.1038/s41434-020-00205-x. Epub ahead of print. PMID: 33149278.

[32] Levy ES, Chang R, Zamecnik CR, Dhariwala MO, Fong L, Desai TA. Multi-Immune Agonist Nanoparticle Therapy Stimulates Type I Interferons to Activate Antigen-Presenting Cells and Induce Antigen-Specific Antitumor Immunity. Mol Pharm. 2021 Feb 4. doi: 10.1021/acs.molpharmaceut.0c00984. Epub ahead of print. PMID: 33541072.

[33] Cooper ZA, Reuben A, Austin-Breneman J, Wargo JA. Does It MEK a Difference? Understanding Immune Effects of Targeted Therapy. Clin Cancer Res. 2015 Jul 15;21(14):3102-4. doi: 10.1158/1078-0432.CCR-15-0363. Epub 2015 May 29. PMID: 26025561; PMCID: PMC4506225.

[34] Biteghe FAN, Chalomie NET, Mungra N, Vignaux G, Gao N, Vergeade A, Okem A, Naran K, Ndong JC, Barth S. Antibody-Based Immunotherapy: Alternative Approaches for the Treatment of

Metastatic Melanoma. Biomedicines. 2020 Sep 3;8(9):327. doi: 10.3390/biomedicines8090327. PMID: 32899183; PMCID: PMC7555584

[35] Yeon M, Kim Y, Jung HS, Jeoung D. Histone Deacetylase Inhibitors to Overcome Resistance to Targeted and Immuno Therapy in Metastatic Melanoma. Front Cell Dev Biol. 2020 Jun 17;8:486. doi: 10.3389/fcell.2020.00486. PMID: 32626712; PMCID: PMC7311641.

[36] Kelly ZR, Gorantla VC, Davar D. The Role of Neoadjuvant Therapy in Melanoma. Curr Oncol Rep. 2020 Jun 29;22(8):80. doi: 10.1007/s11912-020-00944-5. PMID: 32601947.

Chapter 2

Uveal Melanoma

Kristina Horkovicova and Alena Furdova

Abstract

Currently, melanoma of uvea is the most well-known essential tumor, which is intaocular and malignant. Treatment using radiation has now supplanted enucleation as the therapy of decision. Radioactive eye plaques and treatment using proton are being the two most examined radiotherapeutic modalities. All the more as of late, stereotactic radiosurgery and fractionated stereotactic radiotherapy have risen as promising, non-intrusive medicines for uveal melanoma. Technique called stereotactic radiosurgery might be viewed as like "not surgery" on the grounds no extractions are included. All things being equal, it is a serious strategy for radiation treatment that conveys high dosages of radiation to exceptionally little territories and volumes.

Keywords: intraocular tumor, uveal melanoma, radiotherapy, stereotactic radiosurgery

1. Introduction

Malignant melanoma of uvea (iris, ciliary body, and choroid), is the most widely recognized essential intraocular danger in grown-ups. Uveal melanoma (UM) is analyzed generally in more established age, with a dynamically increasing age-explicit frequency rate that tops close to the age of seventy. Ocular melanoma is probably going to metastasize in different lregions of the body, for example, breast, lung, kidney or liver.

There are many factors associated with the development of uveal melanoma. The most important includc gcnctic factors, racc, color of thc cycs, fair coloring of thc skin and the ability to tan. Many observational studies up to date have attempted to explore the relationship between sunlight exposure and risk of uveal melanoma development [1].

Usually, uveal melanomas are in early stages of their development completely asymptomatic. The comparatively low incidence of iris melanomas (anterior segment melanoma) has been attributed to the characteristic features of these tumors. Iris melanomas also rarely metastasize. Posterior melanoma - choroidal melanoma is the most common ocular melanoma type. This type is involved in over 75% of all intraocular melanomas. Iris melanoma wchis is in anterior segment is cytologically less malignant and metastatize less frequently tnak posterios uveal melanomas.

Ordinarily, choroidal melanoma is brown colored, raised mass, and the level of its pigmentation can go from dim earthy colored to thoroughly white, amelanotic.

In advanced stages the symptoms are dependent on tumor location. The most important test to establish the presence of intraocular melanoma, is the examination by an experienced clinician at specialized Ophthalmology Department. Diagnostic testing can be extremely valuable in establishing and confirming the diagnosis.

Prognosis can be influenced by number of factors. The most important are the histopathologic type of cells, the size of tumor, tumor volume, the margins of the tumor, karyotype and grading and staging by TNM Classification (e.g. extraocular extension). Cell type, however, remains the most often used predictor of outcome with genetic results.

The treatment relies upon the site of birthplace (choroid, ciliary body or iris), the size, volume and area of the injury, the general statis of the patient, age of the patient and whether extraocular attack, repeat or metastasis has happened. Extraocular augmentation, repeat, and metastasis are related with a very helpless guess and long - term endurance cannot be normal [2].

Elective therapy modalities have been proposed as of late including extremist careful evacuation of the eye globe (enucleation), nearby resection, light procedures: plaque brachytherapy, charged-molecule radiotherapy, stereotactic photon bar illumination treatment or in start of the tumor transpupillary thermotherapy and photodynamic treatment.

Over the past 3–4 decades diagnostic methods have improved and radiotherapy (external beam, charged particle or brachytherapy) has become the preferred treatment for most of the patients with uveal melanoma. The aim of the treatment is to improve survival and preserve eye globe anatomically with aim to preserve the best vision in patients with uveal melanoma. Different radiation modalities are currently in use in treatment of posterior uveal melanoma in many Ophthalmology Centers. One of the methods of "conservative" approach is the stereotactic radiosurgery (SRS) by linear accelerator [2–5].

2. Uvea and uveal tumors

The uveal parcel frames the center layer (or "vasculo-strong" coat) mass of the eyeball. Uvea layer is a combination of veins, pigmented cells and muscles, woven together by connective tissue. It has a nutritive capacity of the eye globe. The uveal parcel comprises of three anatomical parts, all profoundly vascular and pigmented. The noticeable part in front is the iris (part of the foremost portion of the eye) and it makes the shade of the eye globe. The iris consolidates in reverse into the ciliary body, and the ciliary body offers path to the choroid, to the back fragment of the eye globe, which is such a vascular undercoat between the sclera and the shade retina. It is substantial pigmented, along these lines engrossing light which has gone through the retina.

2.1 Uvea layer

The pigmented cells (the melanocytes) - are derived from the neural crests which have migrated to the skin and mucous membranes. Melanocytes synthesize a special organelle called a melanosome – this is responsible for the characteristic color of the skin in different races. Melanosis (melanocytosis) refers to increased pigmentation caused by hyperplasia or hypertrophy of melanocytes.

Changes in melanocytes usually cause melanomas. Melanocytes produce melanin, which is responsible for skin and hair tone. It can show up on ordinary skin or it might start as a mole or other territory that has changed in appearance. A few moles that are available upon entering the world may form into melanomas during the adulthood.

Benign tumor composed of nevus cells or melanocytes is nevus. In nevi cells contain melanosomes and are therefore capable of producing pigment melanin [1].

2.2 Uveal melanoma

Melanoma is a malignant tumor resulting from a transformation of melanocytes or nevus cells. It may be pigmented or non-pigmented. Melanoma is caused mainly by intense, occasional UV exposure (frequently leading to sunburn), especially in those who are genetically predisposed to the disease. Most melanomas are dark or earthy colored, however they can likewise be skin-shaded, pink, red, purple, blue or white. In the event that melanoma is perceived and treated early, it is quite often reparable, however on the off chance that it is not, the tumor can progress and spread to different pieces of the body, particularly liver, where it turns out to be difficult to treat and can be deadly. Melanomas frequently metastasize widely and the regional lymph nodes, liver, lungs and brain are likely to be involved.

Intraocular melanoma is the most common primary ocular malignant tumor in adults and develops from uvea. Intraocular tumors might be benign or malignant.

Intraocular melanoma is a quite rare type of tumor and it occurs most often in elderly people. There is lot of cases when ophthalmologists detected intraocular melanoma during a routine eye examination. The chance of recovery is depending on factors such as the size, localization and cell type of the tumor. Extraocular extension is the term used to describe the intraocular melanoma which spreads to the optic nerve or nearby tissue of the eye socket and is the sign of the advanced stage of the tumor [6].

Intraocular melanoma of the ciliary body and choroid (structures together called the posterior uvea), is the most common primary ocular malignant tumor in adults. Iris melanomas are a subset of uveal melanomas that tend to have a more benign course, in comparison with posterior uveal melanomas. Anterior segment melanomas have a lower incidence of metastases when compared to ciliary body and choroidal melanomas. Anterior segment melanomas account for about 15% of all uveal melanomas. The incidence of uveal melanoma increases with age and reaches a maximum between the 6th and 7th decade of life. It is more common in males and is uncommon or rare in kids and darker looking people. Uveal melanomas are infrequently two-sided. Be that as it may, the quantity of patients with two-sided inclusion is more noteworthy than would be anticipated by chance alone, subsequently inferring a potential hereditary inclination.

As mentioned before, choroidal melanoma represents the most common primary intraocular tumor in adults. Peak incidence is in the early 60s representing about 7.5 cases per one million populations. Incidence is rare in younger adults under 30 years of age with an estimated peak incidence of about six cases per one hundred million. Caucasians are 8 times more likely to develop the melanoma than Africans or Afro-Americans and 3 times more likely than Asians. Intraocular melanoma is arising from choroid in more than 75% of all the cases. Whether some environmental exposure triggers the development of uveal melanoma remains an open question. Sunlight has been proposed as an environmental risk factor for melanoma generally. Unlike cutaneous melanoma, incidence rates for uveal melanoma have not increased over time and last decades and it does not vary by latitude [7, 8].

2.3 Diagnostic method of uveal melanoma

The first step to diagnose uveal melanoma is patient's history. Patients with uveal melanoma may present with complaints of visual acuity reduction, but many can be without symptoms and the condition is discovered on routine ocular examination or by glasses prescription. In eyes with clear optic media, the diagnosis of posterior uveal melanoma can be made by indirect ophthalmoscopy.

a. ophthalmoscopy, fundus photography,

b. transillumination,

c. perimetry,

d. fluorescein angiography, indocyanine green angiography,

e. ultrasonography (A and B modes),

f. ultrasound biomicroscopy - UBM,

g. optical coherence tomography - OCT,

h. computed tomography - CT,

i. magnetic resonance imaging - MRI,

j. fine-needle biopsy

k. whole body PET/CT to distinguish metastasis.

Depending on their site of growth, posterior uveal melanomas differ in their symptoms, clinical presentation and appearance. A ciliary body melanoma can attain a large size, volume, before it is clinically recognized. It can be seen in association with one or more dilated episcleral blood vessels, it can present itself as an epibulbar pigmented lesion if there is transscleral extension of the tumor. Also, cataract, and/or lens subluxation or secondary glaucoma due to infiltration of the trabecular meshwork in the angle of the eye can be present. The tumor can be envisioned clinically through a broadly enlarged understudy by cut light assessment as an arch formed collection in the area or it can have a diffuse circumferential development design known as "ring melanoma". It can develop anteriorly into the front chamber – iridocorneal point and iris (iridociliary melanoma) or back into the choroid (ciliochoroidal melanoma).

A melanoma of choroid ordinarily presents as a sessile or curve formed collection arranged under the retina. Initial step analytic techniques can be aberrant ophthalmoscopy, ultrasound and fluorescein angiography. Surface orange color at the degree of the retinal shade epithelium can be imagined clinically, particularly in more modest back melanomas. Retinal separations can be seen auxiliary to the tumor development just as Bruch membrane rupture (cellar layer bellow the retinal shade epithelium). We can divide melanoma of chodoid into two groups the first is melanoma with pigment and the second one is melanoma withou pigment and can likewise accept a spread development design with just negligible tumor diameter under 3 mm.

Melanoma of ciliary body and melanomas of choroidea may develop cataracts, extraocular extension, secondary glaucoma. Orbital infiltration can be seen usually when the tumor has large volume, higher stage and they therefore have a worse prognosis [9].

Due to the huge range of clinical, morphologic and cytological changes and an absence of discrete stages it is hard to foresee clinical result in singular instances of uveal melanoma based on intraocular tumor size. His size and volume is perhaps the best boundary used to foresee metastatic infection.

A little tumor - melanoma - is characterized as estimating 3 mm or less in thickness and under 10 mm in breadth because of TNM plot. A tumor is delegated medium-sized in the event that it measures between 3 to 5 mm in thickness and between 10 to 15 mm in width. A huge tumor is more prominent than 5 mm in thickness and in excess of 15 mm in breadth.

Patients, who are diagnosed with a primary choroidal "intraocular" melanoma, have usually no signs or symptoms of metastatic tumor. Even with total body positron emission tomography/computed tomography (PET/CT) imaging, very few patients are found to have their melanomas spread to other parts of their body. Others may be found to have metastasis over the following years. The overall percentage of the patients diagnosed for choroidal melanoma does not develop metastatic melanoma. The size of the tumor is one of the very important factors to predict the risk for metastatic spreading. Treatments that limit tumors ability to enlarge will decrease the chance of metastasis because removing the eye tumor is the best method to prevent future spread from that tumor. It is very important for the patients to have periodic general medical examinations because the treatment itself does not affect micrometastasis that can be already present at the time the treatment occurs.

Patients who have metastatic choroidal melanoma, as mentioned above, seem to have no symptoms. For this reason, they should have periodic medical examinations, physical examinations, blood tests and radiographic imaging tests as X-ray, MRI, CT or PET/CT. Later on, patients may have symptoms like loss of their appetite, difficulty with breathing or fatigue.

The highest percentage of metastatic choroidal melanoma is likely to be found in the liver. Metastases in this area of the body can be discovered by blood tests or abdominal imaging studies even in cases when patients are asymptomatic. Besides this, other organs also can be affected, e.g. subcutaneous lymph nodes, lung, bone and brain. A needle biopsy can be used to aspirate tumor cells for cytopathologic examination, when a liver or skin metastasis is suspected.

The liver is the known site of metastasing of choroidal melanoma. Hepatic enzyme levels are tested in all patients with melanoma of uvea. The most sensitive tests of liver capacity are serum antacid phosphate levels, glutamate oxaloacetic transaminase, lactate dehydrogenase and gamma-glutamyl transpeptidase. These test results are negative at closure hour in the majority of patients with choroidal melanoma. If any of the results of these research devices is anomalous, ultrasonography and CT of the liver are displayed. Both imaging modalities have low susceptibility to metastases with a diameter of less than 10–20 mm [10–13].

2.4 Survival modeling of intraocular melanoma

Endurance displaying gives a sign of guess. Likewise, it empowers exceptional measures to be focused just as it improves the assessment of clinical methodology.

Endurance rates give a more precise system so as to depict the visualization for patients with a specific stage and type of disease. These rates are frequently founded on past results of huge quantities of individuals who had the sickness, however they cannot anticipate what will occur in a specific patient's case. In patients whose malignancy is bound to the eye, the five-year endurance rate is about 80%. This is as opposed to melanomas that have spread to inaccessible pieces of the body, where the five-year endurance rate is about 15%.

2.4.1 Prognostic factors for uveal melanoma

Pigmented choroidal lessions that are somewhat raised might be called vague sores and present a test concerning determination and the board. Given the dangers and restrictions regarding getting histological affirmation of harm, ophthalmologists need to depend on clinical qualities recognized as prescient of development and metastasis so as to separate little melanomas from raised choroidal melanocytic tumors that are likely kindhearted. Shields et al. distinguished five components related with danger of development of little choroidal melanocytic lessions under 3 mm in diameter using examinations retrospectively of around 1300 patients [14].

These factors were:

1. posterior tumor margin touching the disc;

2. visual symptoms;

3. tumor thickness bigger than 2.0 mm;

4. subretinal fluid;

5. orange pigment.

In 4 percent of patients was observed growth of lesion with none of risk factor, in 36 percent of patients was present one risk factor, and three or more factors were present in more than 50 percent of patients.

Clinical factors associated with an increased risk of metastasis included:

1. growth documentation;

2. increased tumor diameter (bigger than/equal to 1.1 mm);

3. posterior margin touching the disc.

The small-tumor observational study conducted by the COMS Group identified similar risk factors associated with tumor growth; namely

1. apical tumor thickness was greater,

2. initial basal diameter was larger,

3. orange pigment was present,

4. there were no drusen,

5. retinal pigment epithelial change adjacent to the tumor was absent.

Prognostic factors for uveal melanoma can be subdivided into three categories: clinical, histopathological and genetical. Clinical predictive factors have been extensively described. Location of the tumor, its thickness and diameter are clinical factors predicting tumor growth. In addition, age at time of treatment, male gender and secondary glaucoma were prognostic relevant. Shields constructed a mnemonic "TFSOM" "to find small ocular melanoma" (thickness greater than 2 mm, subretinal fluid, symptoms, orange pigment and margin at the disc) to assist in identifying small choroidal melanoma at risk for growth. The most important histopathological markers predicting clinical behavior are the presence of epithelioid cells, largest tumor diameter, sclera invasion, and presence of vascular loops. Other valuable prognostic factors are the presence of mitotic figures and tumor-infiltrating lymphocytes. The cell sort of uveal melanoma is identified with guess. Patients with tumors made out of unadulterated axle cells have a more ideal guess, and those with a part of epithelioid cells (blended or epithelioid-cell types) have a more awful visualization. Melanomas with a low mitotic movement show a superior anticipation. Tumor invasion by lymphocytes has been related with diminished endurance [15].

3. Overview of methods of treatment of uveal melanoma

These days there are a lot greater treatment choices other than enucleation, which was the main alternative for a large portion of a century ago. The more moderate treatment choices mean to save the influenced eye and hold vision. Treatment of uveal melanoma relies upon different variables including age of the patients, foundational strength of the patient, state of the contrary eye, tumor size and area.

Nevertheses, metastases cannot be prevented. Based on the theoretical models, clinically manifest metastases are likely to occour 5 or 6 years onset of the systemic dissemination. By the time we diagnosis uveal melanoma, micrometastases may have been spread as of now. Along these lines, metastatic sickness happening after therapy is not unprecedented. Roughly 50% of the patients will kick the bucket from the sickness inside 10 to 15 years of enucleation. When a metastasis is found the endurance is under 7 months. In the event that a metastasis emerges as a lone injury in the liver, expanded endurance might be acquired by nearby resection of the tumor mass.

Tumor area and size are considered to be two of the primary factors in deciding on the treatment of ocular melanoma. There is no reason to save the eye if a small melanoma in a necessary place completely destroyed vision. It is important to remember this - patients who have undergone enucleation and individuals who have undergone radiation treatment respond appropriately when they receive information about the nature of their patients after treatment. The most important for them was tumor endurance.

Treatment using radiation is a typical therapy for intraocular melanoma that utilizes high energy radiation to kill tumor cells. Radiation treatment can regularly safeguard some vision, albeit once in a while this is lost at any rate since radiation harms different pieces of the eye. The structure of the eye is saved and this is mainly the advantage of this sort of treatment.

Radiation treetment can be divided into two categories. External radiation treatment that utilizes a machine outside the body to send radiation toward the tumor, and the second type is inside radiation treatment that utilizes a radioactive substance fixed in needles, seeds, wires, or catheters that are set legitimately into or close to the tumor. The manner in which the radiation treatment is given relies upon the sort and phase of the tumor being dealt with. In ophthalmooncology field we utilize both photon pillar light and furthermore proton beam irradiation.

The metastatic free survival rate, the local control and the late toxicity were studied in patients that underwent fractionated Stereotactic Radiation Therapy (fSRT) for uveal melanoma. These patients had a median follow-up 32 months and were given five fractions of 10 Gy. The results showed that fSRT is an effective treatment for uveal melanoma with a good local control. There were performed 15 enucleations after irradiation mainly because of neurovascular glaucoma [16].

Plaque therapy is the most often utilized framework for delivering radiation The other methods are Gamma Knife or methods that include proton beam. Radiation plaque treatment which offers great tumor control, can frequently safeguard helpful vision, and has a fundamental visualization that is practically identical to that of enucleation. Enucleation remains the standard strategy for the board of the biggest melanomas of the choroid and ciliary body. The Collaborative Ocular Melanoma Study (COMS) is randomized clinical trial assessing essential enucleation versus beam radiation done externaly followed by enucleation in the management of patients with choroidal melanomas. The study demonstrated that the two options to be used in same medium sized tumors. COMS studied also treatment of large tumors and found out that combined external radiotherapy followd by enucleation shown that there is no limit in orbital recurrence of the tumor mass [10–13].

3.1 One day session stereotactic radiosurgery for uveal melanoma: our experience

Stereotactic radiosurgery (SRS) is technically challenging therapeutic irradiating method. SRS complements or supplies (replaces) classic surgical intervention. The purpose of using SRS is single, because high therapeutic irradiation dosage is to involve only an exact specified tumor structure, while the other organs and structures are contemporary protected. We use special hardware equipment of workstation and software. Professional experiences of specialists of various fields (neurosurgeon trained in stereotactic radiosurgery, radiation oncologist, ophthalmologist, radiologist, clinical physicist and registered nurse trained for radiosurgery) are needed.

The surgery is determined by patient preparation before surgery intervention. This consists of processing of health of the patient and whole patients imaging documentation. It is important to analyze the patient's illnesses and the patient's indication by the Indicating Commission (BTB). The Commission consists of the members as a neurosurgeon trained in radiosurgery, radiation oncologists, ophthalmologists, radiologists and clinical physicists. Just after the see the records and imaging of the patients they decides whether to do SRS or not. The Progress Committee selects, on the basis of a recommendation on the suitability of ophthalmic oncological surgery, which evaluates the suitability of conventional surgery, stereotactic radiosurgery, fractional stereotactic radiosurgery, intensity modulated radiotherapy (IMRT) or three-dimensional comfort radiotherapy (3 D-CRT).

Indicated patients for stereotactic radiosurgical intervention are concerned for inpatient care Ophthalmology Department of Faculty of Medicine, Comenius University in Bratislava. The whole hospitalization lasts most often three days. The patient admission includes interview with the patient with detailed information about the course of operation, performance benefits as well as acquaintance with potential acute and late postoperative complications (adverse effects), after the informed consent is signed by the patient.

Patient's affirmation in hospital bed department (clinical care) is carried two days before the surgery. Clinical examination will be done in detail. The documentation patient brought is studied, in case there are some missing examinations they are done and completed by the time of the surgery and a preoperative pharmacotherapy treatment in hospital bed department is placed on. One day before the stereotactic radiosurgery (SRS) patient has to use premedication. Within the preoperative premedication the patient is using the antiedema therapy, which intensity depends on the size, location of the lesion and the presence of edema. The presented therapy continues at the day of surgery and also the following day.

The patient's record must incorporate the age at treatment, volume and size of tumor, the most extreme stature of the tumor estimated by A, B scan ultrasound. The presence and the degree of secondary retinal detachment, and note if there is an extrascleral expansion must be recorded in patients file. Tumor volume, in every patient straightforwardly after computer CT and MRI assessment is determined as the progression of SRS strategy and is included to the scheme of stereotactic planning.

Mechanical fixation to the stereotactic (Leibinger) frame is done before stereotactic irradiation immobilization of the affected eye. Stiches are put under 4 direct extraocular muscles through conjunctiva and through the upper and lower lid. The stereotactic frame is fixed to the head and the stiches are attached to the stereotactic frame on the side of affected eye. The patient undergoes a CT examination with the eye tied to the patient's frame. After fixation and administration of the drug contrast agent, the examination is performed on one-millimeter scans. After completing the CT examination, the patient is transferred to an MRI examination. The patient undergoes an MRI examination with the eye still fixed on a stereotactic frame. After placement in the MRI, a contrast agent is administered. MRI and CT imaging records are sent to a computer console in the computer room.

At that point after the CT and MRI examinations patient is transported to the resting room of Department of radiotherapy of St. Elizabeth Oncological Institute and is waiting for exposure in the linear accelerator.

Clinical physicist processes imaging records for the purpose of fusion and subsequent planning of stereotactic radiosurgery irradiation. By the fusion of images obtained from the CT and MRI it is obtained an accurate image and the structure-relationship of operated patient. CT examination does not always perfect morphology image of targeting and risk structures, but it is an accurate and does not distort the displaying structures. MRI can distort displaying targeted and risk structures, particularly in the area of bone structures arises the distortion. Neural structures are showed in three dimensions, which allows a reconstruction and good distinctiveness of targeted and risk neural structures. Planning system communicates only with the CT imaging, in which information is transmitted from other investigating modalities. Clinical physicist makes by the fusion the correction of the treating volume of a focus and risk structures from the MRI records to CT imaging.

After imaging the target and risk structures, the neurosurgeon draws the target volumes and risk structures in sections of one millimeter in a CT record and consults them with an ophthalmologist and radiologist. The planning of stereotactic treatment after the fusion of CT and MR is optimized according to the critical structures, which are the lens, the optic nerve on both sides, and chiasma is also marked as the critical structure.

The best plan is after applied for therapy at linear accelerator. Calculation of tumor volume depends on the ROI (region of interest) of the tumor and 3D reconstruction is done. The planned therapeutic dose is 35.0 Gy by 99% of DVH (dose volume histogram). Model LINAC C 600 C/D Varian with 6 MeV X is utilized.

3.1.1 Stereotactic planning

The stereotactic treatment arranging after combination of CT and MRI pictures is streamlined by the basic structures - focal point, optic nerve, and furthermore focal point and optic nerve at the contralateral side, chiasm.

The planned therapeutic dose in SRS is 35.0 Gy, TDmin. The dose varies from 35.0 to 38.0 Gy, TDmax 37.0–50.0 Gy to the margin of the lesion. We use PTV (treatment volume planning) at least 95% isodose planning. Doses for critical structures such as the optic nerve and optic disc are less than 8.0 Gy and 10.0 Gy for the anterior segment of the eye (**Figures 1** and **2**).

The clinical physicist embeds the plan into the verification system after printing the radiation parameters and documentation. At the same day after the planning is finished the patient undergoes irradiation at linear accelerator in the afternoon.

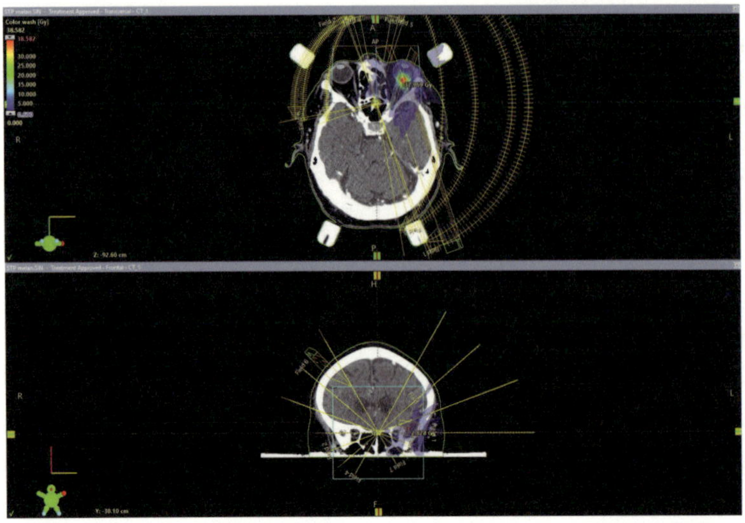

Figure 1.
Stereotactic planning scheme for patient with uveal melanoma on linear accelerator (TD – 35.0 Gy) – Part a. origin: Dept. of stereotactic radiosurgery, Bratislava.

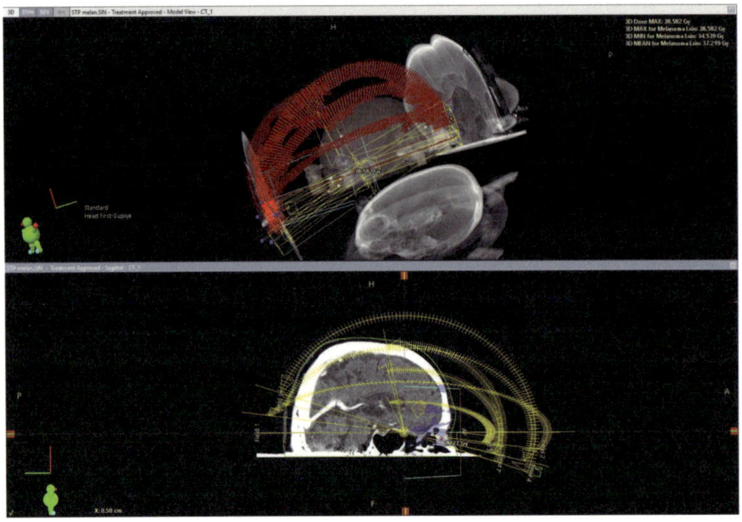

Figure 2.
Stereotactic planning scheme for patient with uveal melanoma on linear accelerator (TD – 35.0 Gy) – Part B. origin: Dept. of stereotactic radiosurgery, Bratislava.

Mechanical fixation to the stereotactic frame ensures that the head while the examination and treatment is in the same, right position. Along with the merger of images from CT and MRI is guaranteed the accuracy of the method in the order of tenths of a millimeter.

When the exposure id completed the patient is unfixed from the operating table and moved into the operating room. According to volume and collimators the whole procedure lasts from 15 to 50 minutes.

In the case of application of stereotactic radiosurgery using micro-multileaf collimator makes clinical physicist verification plan using the verification phantom. He inserts the irradiation plan of patient into verification system of linear accelerator and verifies the accuracy of irradiation plan applications into verification phantom by irradiation of verification phantom by the dosimetric system.

3.1.2 Stereotactic radiosurgery for uveal melanoma: Our results

Treatment of uveal melanoma in Slovakia is performed on direct quickening agent LINAC. One-fraction LINAC radiotherapy/radiosurgery is an unusual approach to treatment of choroidal melanoma. Hypofractionation with a broad shoulder in linear-quadratic model for radioresistant tumors like choroidal melanoma is still in discussion.

We evaluated in our study local failure which leads into enucleation as an end point in patients treated by SRS with long-term follow-up having accrued at the time of analysis. We evaluate in our study the treatment of posterior uveal melanoma by one-day session of LINAC stereotactic radiosurgery.

The first goal of our study was to evaluate treatment BCVA decline in patients who has posterior uveal melanoma treated with SRS in 6 months interval 24 months after SRS.

The second goal was to find out whether the group of patients with better initial visual acuity on the beginning of treatment would have also a better chance to preserve vision. The observed after-treatment decline in BCVA was 24 months interval after the treatment.

The third goal was observation of the tumor regression by the maximum elevation measurement using B-scan ultrasound in the group of patients with single irradiation (SRS) in interval 1 and 2 years after the treatment.

For patients treated by SRS in the period 2001–2008 was a retrospective analysis was undertaken. At the Department of Ophthalmology, Comenius University in Bratislava we reviewed 84 patients records with choroidal melanoma or with ciliary body melanoma treated in this period. 44 patients underwent primary enucleation (52.4%) out of 84 patients and 40 patients underwent SRS as an initial treatment (47.6%). The diagnosis was established on the basic of ophthalmological examination, ultrasound, CT or MRI examination. Excluded from analyzed cohort were metastatic intraocular tumors, juxtapapillary localized tumors and melanocytomas.

Each patient record must have details such as the age at treatment, tumor size, tumor volume, the maximum height of the tumor by A, B scan ultrasound, the presence and the extent of secondary retinal detachment, and if there are signs of extrascleral spread.

The tumors were divided into 3 groups as follows: small up to 4 or 5 mm of maximal elevation, middle 4–8 mm, and large over 8 mm.

In the group of one stereotactic irradiation, an increase in the tumor was observed in a 6-month interval by ultrasound with a B-scan ophthalmologist. We compared tumor regression by measuring maximal elevation using B-scan ultrasound in a group of 25 patients with single irradiation (SRS) at 12 and 24 months post-treatment.

3.1.3 Enucleation versus stereotactic radiosurgery: Our results

We analyzed the treatment outcome and possible survival difference between radical surgical treatment (primary enucleation) and stereotactic radiosurgery (SRS) at the Department of Ophthalmology, Comenius University in Bratislava, in patients with posterior uveal melanoma.

Patients treated for uveal melanoma in posterior during the period 2001–2008 are analyzed in the study. The goal of the study was to compare the relapse-free survival in the cohort of patients initially treated by SRS or they primary underwent enucleation. Together we included 84 patients. Treatment was determined on a case-by-case basis.

We analyzed each patient's record with ciliary body or choroidal melanoma treated by enucleation. We divided them into two groups: first group had 44 patients (52%) using surgical treatment and the second group had 40 patients (48%) using SRS treatment. The therapeutic attitude was set up based on ophthalmoscopy, ultrasound (A, B mode), other ophthalmological findings, visual acuity, and general status of each patient and MRI examination. Volume of the tumor was determined by using the formula:

$$\text{Tumor volume} = \frac{\pi}{6} * \text{length} * \text{width} * \text{height} \qquad (1)$$

$$\text{Td} = \frac{0{,}30103 * \text{number of months}}{\log_{10}(\text{final volume}) - \log_{10}(\text{starting volume})} \qquad (2)$$

The disease-free interval was defined as the period from treatment (either enucleation or SRS) until the development of metastasis, or the death of the patient. The patients after enucleation were examined by ophthalmologist every six months, with a monthly interval in the first six months, dependent on problems with using individual prosthesis. The patients after stereotactic radiosurgery were examined by an ophthalmologist every three months: visual acuity, biomicroscopy (slit lamp), intraocular pressure, ultrasound in A and B mode, fundus photography and since the year 2007 also OCT (optical coherence tomography) was routinely done. Post radiation complications and tumor dimension and extent of secondary retinal detachment were observed. The patients were observed in the period from 2001 (01/01) to 2008 (31/12) and the data were analyzed.

The disease-free interval was defined as the time from treatment until the development of metastases. Patients were seen in three months interval in the first year after the SRS, later in six months interval following SRS. Patients in both groups were regularly in six months interval recommended to their oncologist to a liver ultrasound, abdominal ultrasound, liver function test, brain CT, chest X-ray to confirm or exclude the presence of metastases. In individual cases they were recommended to brain CT or PET/CT.

In the period 2001–2008 a total number of 84 patients with intermediate or large uveal melanoma were treated with either radical surgical removal of the whole eyeball (enucleation), or SRS. In a group of 40 patients who underwent SRS there were 22 male and 18 female - the total median age was 55 years; the median age of female was 54 years and 58 years of male. In a group of 44 patients with enucleated eyes the median age was 68.5 year. In the group there were 21 males (median age 64), and 23 females (median age 73). The median tumor volume in group of ste reotactic patients was 0,65 cm^3 (0,4 - 0,8), in group of enucleated patients 1,1 cm^3 (0,8 - 1,25).

Five patients treated in the first step with SRS required subsequent enucleation due to the complications - secondary neovascular glaucoma. Three patients of this subgroup underwent pars plana vitrectomy with endoresection of the tumors plus silicon oil, but the enucleation was necessary due to the complication - relapse of the tumor.

Histopathologically in the group of enucleated eyes after SRS due to complications in four patients with malignant melanoma of the mixed cell type, in two cases an epithelioid type, and in one case a spindle-cell type A was confirmed.

In the group of primary enucleated eyes, there were four findings of an epithelioid-cell type, one case of a nodular type, as well as 10 cases of both, a mixed-cell type and 29 cases of a spindle-cell type (A or B) melanoma.

The age and tumor volume are important explanatory variables (termed covariates) that are assumed to be associated with survival and need to be incorporated in the model. Results on logistic regression confirmed significance of the model with the predictors age and tumor volume (P = 0.01). The tumor volume was a significant unique predictor (P = 0.035); age with its borderline probability value of 0.1 could be assumed as possibly associated with the outcome. The estimator of survival rates adjusted for these predictors was constructed based on Cox's regression model which examines the relationship between survival and both predictors.

3.1.4 Complications after stereotactic radiosurgery: Our results

The fundamental objective of radioactive therapy is to control malignancy while maintaining useful vision. Present techniques result in a high incidence of tumor control for intermediate and small lesions (< 8 mm in height). Tumor control for enormous sores is not ideal, also, here is a higher frequency of late complexities bringing about hindered vision in huge sores. All things considered, radiation portion decrease to the uninvolved piece of the eye will lessen the rate of late difficulties while keeping up a high occurrence of tumor control for more modest tumors.

Utilizing of 3-D radiation dosimetry is accepted that will have significant advantage as far as therapy enhancement and lower frequency of late inconveniences. Such a 3-D framework grants exact pre-treatment arranging and adjustments of the arrangement at short notification, for example, on account of new intraoperative discoveries. There is overpowering proof that threatening melanoma of the uveal plot can be dealt with securely with radioactive plaques with long haul endurance rates equivalent to those of enucleation. We think, that the vessels around the optic plate are harmed by full portion light, prompting retinal ischemia, and this courtesies the presence of neovascular glaucoma. Safeguarding of the eye work is normal in most of radioactive-plaque treatment treated patients. Utilization of low energy isotopes, collimation of individual seeds, and routine utilization of 3-D imaging and 3-D dosimetry should assist with promoting improve episcleral plaque treatment. In writing the rate of post-radiotherapy enucleation from all causes is about 20%. The diminishing of the occurrence of intricacies as waterfall, radiation papillitis, radiation maculopathy, optional glaucoma is because of extremely exacting signs of back uveal melanoma. Today, no randomized planned investigation of the impact of the elective moderate medicines for choroidal melanoma on visual result have been performed.

In our group of patients after Ru106/Rh106 plaque treatment the accompanying late intricacies prompted crumbling of visual keenness and were seen at the last subsequent assessment:

- macular pulverization due to scarring around the tumor, optic nerve decay,
- macular degeneration, retinopathy, fractional focal point haziness, complete waterfall, glassy discharge, optional glaucoma, apoplexy of the focal retinal vein.

The patient will develop radiation cataract if more than 30% of the periphery of the lens is irradiated. If the diameter of the tumor is large, invasion of the iris may occur, or if the anterior margin of the tumor is well in front of the equator, the lens may be more sensitive to irradiation. Post-radiation cataracts can occur even if less than 30% of its periphery is irradiated.

Our clinical experience shows that auxiliary enucleation after stereotactic radiosurgery because of light neuropathy and optional glaucoma was essential just in 11.5% in 3 to 5 years stretch after illumination.

3.1.5 Follow-up

The patient after SRS is controlled regularly ambulatory, the clinical and MRI examinations are carried out, which are made ambulatory, initially and MRI is controlled after 3 months after SRS, first year, next two years in half yearly intervals, then 1 time a year in a following 5 years. Patient is monitored by an ophthalmologist in 2 weeks, later 6 weeks and 3 months interval - visual acuity, intraocular pressure, slit lamp examination, fundus photo, ultrasound – B-scan, OCT, perimetry. In 3-months' interval patient is send to MRI control [2, 17, 18].

4. Discussion

Fifty years back, enucleation was the main acknowledged choice of treatment for melanoma, perception until recorded development was supported for little tumors that could not be unquestionably analyzed as melanomas on beginning introduction. These days with the openness and showed sufficiency of eyeball-sparing medicines, a conflict can be made for before treatment of these vague lessions. Data from the COMS primers reveals that melanoma-related mortality varies with tumor size at period of treatment. For medium estimated tumors (portrayed as tumors 2.5 to 10 mm in apical height and up to 16 mm in greatest basal width), melanoma-express mortality was 10% at five years, and 18% at 10 years. For huge tumors (those astounding the size models for medium tumors in either apical height or greatest basal expansiveness; or peripapillary tumors with an apical height more conspicuous than 8 mm), the rates extended to generally 27% at five years and 40% at 10 years. Also, as referenced above, archived development before treatment has been demonstrated to be a danger factor for metastasis. In any case, development might be a marker for more forceful tumors, and it has not been demonstrated that treating these tumors prior diminishes mortality [7].

Our present strategies for radiotherapy consider powerful nearby tumor control with eyeball preservation, yet visual morbidity is still high. In this manner, it is important to gauge the mortality hazard caused via cautious perception before treatment of uncertain sores against the outcomes of visual misfortune actuated by treatment.

In a small COMS tumor observation study, there were six melanoma-related transitions from a cohort of 67 tumor patients treated after baseline perception. Only two of these transitions occurred within five years of enrollment, resulting in an inaccurate five-year death rate with an explicit melanoma of 3% [11].

One-portion LINAC radiotherapy/radiosurgery is an abnormal way to deal with treatment of choroidal melanoma. Hypofractionation with a wide shoulder in straight quadratic model is still in conversation for radioresistant tumors like choroidal melanoma. In this examination we assessed nearby disappointment prompting enucleation as an end point in patients treated by SRS with long haul development having accumulated at the hour of investigation [19].

Picture combination of a differentiation improved attractive reverberation imaging (MRI) and figured tomography (CT) is utilized for treatment arranging co-ordinates. A few creators incline toward light before enucleation for huge uveal melanoma. This treatment is utilized in a method of SRS with a solitary division managed with a valuable spatial exactness utilizing a collimating framework.

Because of our outcomes the saw after-treatment decrease in BCVA was not emphatically connected with higher pervasiveness of better BCVA before SRS, however the anatomical outcome after the treatment was at any rate anatomically saved eyeball [17].

Empowering our outcomes legitimize further examinations to assess one day meeting method and its viability as an option in contrast to other light helpful methodologies. On the off chance that we utilized single SRS treatment just, in patients with tumor volume over 0.6 cm^3 the danger of relapse was high, over half and extra treatment was essential. As per our experience the portion of 35.0 Gy is not adequate light and may cause backslide just in patients with high volume tumors, over 0.6 cm^3. By breaking down individual patient's consequences of this examination, we presume that this treatment is adequate for little and middle of the road tumors with the rise not more than 6 mm, resp. volume up to 0.4 cm^3 as per individual stereotactic arranging plan of every patient as a solitary treatment system. Auxiliary enucleation after stereotactic radiosurgery due to mild neuropathy and secondary glaucoma was vital in only 11.5% at 3 to 5 years after illumination. In our examination, proximal tumor control was effective in 95% of patients at 3 years after stereotactic radiosurgery and in 85% of patients at 5 years after stereotactic radiosurgery [20].

As indicated by our outcomes one-day session SRS with 35.0 Gy is adequate to treat little and center stage melanoma. No endurance distinction inferable from stereotactic light or consolidated and surgical attitude - enucleation of uveal melanoma has been exhibited in the review concentrate in Slovak Republic. Enucleation after SRS in 7 patients was in stretch 6 months to two years after SRS. A little distinction is conceivable, yet a clinically significant contrast in death rates, regardless of whether from all causes or from metastatic melanoma, is improbable.

A high degree of local control can be achieved with a five-year control rate exceeding 95% in patients treated with charged particles. Radiotherapy with a 62 MeV proton rod with a cyclotron achieves a high rate of close tumor control and visual protection, with the visual outcome depending on the size and area of the tumor.

Huge, imminent, randomized preliminaries were intended to look at mortality figures for medium-sized melanomas treated by brachytherapy or enucleation. The outcomes could not show the distinction in death rates between the two treatment bunches following a limit of 12 years of development.

In the most recent years, the administration of patients with uveal melanoma has changed toward eyeball saving strategies. Options other than extreme enucleation range from perception to perception to transpupillary thermotherapy, block-extraction, endoresection with standards plana vitrectomy, brachytherapy utilizing an assortment of radioisotopes, outside bar radiotherapy, charged particles and stereotactic radiosurgery or strategies can be approached. SRS has recently been proposed as an optional treatment for posterior uveal melanoma. Treatment for each patient should be selected according to the patient's general condition, stage and nature of the tumor. COMS is planned to provide remote information on regular history as well as a useful speech.

Single-division stereotactic radiosurgery is normally finished with a Gamma Knife just as more as of late with a CyberKnife. The remedial single portion has been diminished to as low as 35.0 Gy in the course of recent years without decrease in tumor control. Dosages of 40.0 Gy conveyed at the half isodose bring about great nearby tumor control and satisfactory harmfulness. Since radiobiological contemplates show a potential favorable position of hypo fractionated treatment over a solitary huge portion to clean uveal melanoma cell lines, fractionated stereotactic radiotherapy (SRT) has increased extra interest. Other than expanded tumor control, poisonousness ought to hypothetically be diminished by fractionation.

Direct quickening agents (LINAC) have the upside of an attainable fractionation. Most LINAC contemplates utilize a hypo fractionated plan of 4–5 portions and complete dosages somewhere in the range of 50.0 and 70.0 Gy. The viability of SRT for uveal melanoma has been demonstrated in various investigations with neighborhood tumor control rates announced over 90%, 5 and 10 years after treatment. Radiogenic results after SRT are accounted for also to different types of radiotherapy, with waterfall advancement, radiation retinopathy, opticopathy and neovascular glaucoma being liable for most of optional vision misfortunes and auxiliary enucleations. Generally speaking, stereotactic photon bar radiotherapies (SRS and SRT) are viewed as compelling treatment modalities for uveal melanoma, with promising late tumor control and poisonousness rates. SRS is a generally new strategy, so there is a requirement for multi-focus preliminary to contrast the results following stereotactic radiosurgery and different techniques. Nonetheless, as of recently, no investigation has been acted in this point. Studies contrasting endurance rates following enucleation versus more current treatment modalities, including SRS, recommended comparative rates for tantamount sores and in light of the fact that revealed nearby tumor control rate following SRS seem similar, we offer SRS to patients who might somehow or another require enucleation [1].

Stereotactic photon treatment of uveal melanoma, in light of CT and MRI pictures, is a protected and exact treatment choice. Neighborhood control was discovered to be superb. Due to choice models, the quantity of patients in the investigation with decreased visual sharpness will likely expansion later on.

Neighborhood power over 95% shows up in certain investigations: in the investigation of Dieckmann nearby control is 98% after a middle perception time 33 months follow up. The perception time is still too short to even consider allowing complete ends, yet their outcomes are tantamount with the 82–98% nearby control rate detailed by different gatherings after a middle perception season of as long as 15 years [21].

Visual misfortune after proton pillar light was depicted in 33–47% following 1 and 2 years, individually, for tumors situated close to the optic plate and fovea.

Different creators announced in a review study that light of 30.0 Gy of in excess of 2 mm of the optic nerve head started an optic neuropathy.

In the investigation of Dieckmann because of troublesome tumor size and area in the region of basic structures, for example optic nerve and macula, visual decrease was seen in a high number of the patients. After a perception season of beyond what a half year visual sharpness can be assessed in 79 patients. In the gathering of 77 patients 85.5% gave visual sharpness of 0.1 or better before radiotherapy. LINAC based stereotactic light for melanoma of uvea is plausible and all around endured. Can be offered to patients with medium measured and horribly found melanoma of uvea who are looking for an eye-protecting therapy [22].

To accomplish great visual keenness result it is significant right limitation of the tumor. Brachytherapy Ru106 of back choroidal melanoma accomplishes great preservation of vision if the tumor does not stretch out near the optic nerve or fovea. Realize that the intensity of a test to look at endurance in at least two gatherings is connected not to the all out example size but rather to the quantity of functions of interest, (for example, passing for this situation). At the end of the day, the endurance tests perform better when the editing is not excessively substantial, and, specifically, when the example of controlling is comparable over the various gatherings. High number of right-blue-penciled information (from those patients who actually were alive toward the finish of perception, or exited the investigation for different reasons other than death before its end) could influence the unwavering quality of the outcomes. Subsequently, the substantial controlling may confuse the assessment of the endurance model, since it diminishes the comparable number of subjects uncovered (in danger) at later occasions, decreasing the successful example sizes. Also, little example sizes may additionally expand the impact of the presumption infringement. It is not sensible, notwithstanding, to drop the chose informative variable(s) from the model, since there are "genuine world" reasons why these specific factors ought to stay in the last model [23].

To this date, no preliminary examination of the dosimetry, safety and viability of SRS or evaluation of gamma knife radiosurgery results for melanoma has been performed. So far information from several reported cases recommends that SRS can have comparable close tumor control rates, metastases, death rates and involvement rates brachytherapy. Late examinations recommend that gamma knife radiosurgery and SRS may be an appropriate choice for the treatment of uveal melanoma in those patients in whom ulcers are not suitable for conventional brachytherapy. The findings in the setting recommend a part of SRS in the treatment of selected cases of uveal melanoma [24].

Entanglements after specific techniques can prompt auxiliary neovascular glaucoma and may result to the enucleation, that is the reason the eye maintenance is one of the fundamental objectives of the moderate treatment. A multivariate information investigation by utilizing the directed learning methods, specifically the calculation known as Regularized Least Squares (RLS) was utilized in investigation of Mosci. Their examination was the biggest one in Italy and they exhibited the brilliant neighborhood tumor control, endurance and eye consistency standard after the proton shaft light treatment. As their results suggest, further improvements in treatment delivery may be important in determining visual outcomes and complexities after proton shaft therapy in visual melanoma dosing and delivery [25].

The basic problems of radiotherapy in one meeting are the effects of propagation and hypofractionation of the part. The size and area of the tumor, for example closer than 2 mm from the optical plate, are the main components for determining the clinical evaluation of the visual acuity result.

Distinguishing proof of danger variables may lessen the paces of repeat and lead to less inconveniences, safeguarding of the eye, improved visual capacity and, conceivably, better endurance result. Repeat of optic neuropathy after stereotactic radiosurgery is an issue by intraocular tumors as well as for example by perichiasmal tumors stereotactic illumination. Albeit uncommon, optic neuropathy may follow radiosurgery to injuries close to the visual pathways. Cautious portion arranging guided by MRI with limitation of the maximal portion to the visual pathways to under 8.0 Gy will probably diminish the frequency of this entanglement.

Similar issues with visual sharpness misfortune as in stereotactic radiosurgery are found in patients after other radiotherapy methods, for example brachytherapy. In the sequential arrangement of patients after Ru106 brachytherapy, patients held some helpful vision in the principal postoperative years and a couple even improved visual sharpness, notwithstanding, the drawn out visual result is poor with a proceeding with visual keenness misfortune over the long run. Countless patients became visually impaired or lost perusing capacity following 5 years, either due to radiation confusions or auxiliary enucleation.

Stereotactic radiosurgery and fractionated stereotactic radiotherapy have developed as promising, non-intrusive medicines for uveal melanoma [26]. Albeit, verifiably, melanoma has been viewed as a moderately radioresistant tumor, fresher information have tested this perspective, and radiation treatment is currently viewed as a helpful segment of the restorative armamentarium for harmful melanoma. As indicated by our outcomes a solitary one-day meetings SRS with 35.0 Gy is adequate to treat little and center stage melanoma. No endurance distinction inferable from stereotactic light or joined and careful mentality - enucleation of uveal melanoma has been exhibited in the review concentrate in Slovakia.

In our examination bunches researched, endurance investigation changed for indicators demonstrated that the gathering of patients after stereotactic radiosurgery had similar result as the gathering of patients treated with extremist medical procedure. In light of our examination, we expect that the endurance guess is basically dictated by the personality of the tumor in relationship to the status of the patient. Clinically, the main factors that influence the metastatic cycle are the limitation and size (volume) of the sore.

There has been played out no multicenter preliminary to survey dosimetry, wellbeing and adequacy of SRS, or to assess results of gamma knight radiosurgery for melanoma yet, yet information from a few announced case arrangement recommend that SRS could have comparative nearby tumor control rate, metastasis rate, death rate and intricacies rate when contrasted with brachytherapy. Late investigations have proposed that gamma knight radiosurgery and SRS might be a fitting option for treating uveal melanoma in those patients, in whom sores are ineligible for customary brachytherapy. The discoveries in the arrangement propose a part of SRS in the treatment of chose instances of uveal melanoma. Treatment by either essential enucleation or SRS as per our outcomes does not seem to impact the improvement of metastases in patients with uveal melanoma; the endurance anticipation is basically controlled by the stage and character of the tumor.

No endurance contrast inferable from stereotactic light or extremist careful disposition - enucleation of uveal melanoma has been shown in this review study. A little contrast is conceivable, yet a clinically significant distinction in death rates, regardless of whether from all causes or from metastatic melanoma, is far-fetched. SRS is a non-intrusive option in contrast to enucleation in the treatment of uveal melanoma with a high tumor control. There is a requirement for multi-focus preliminaries to think about the results following stereotactic radiosurgery in treatment of uveal melanoma.

5. Conclusion

The single light of the tumor itself is another methodology – it has been appeared to accomplish ultrasonic tumor relapse along these lines to brachytherapy. SRS of extracerebral sores like uveal melanoma has been developed over the most recent twenty years and is an elective treatment for center and enormous back choroidal melanoma. With plaque radiotherapy, eye rescue is accomplished, and especially for cases in which the tumor is found away from the optic circle or macula, helpful vision can be held after treatment.

As indicated by the creators experience dependent on consequences of their exploration aftereffects of the adequacy of LINAC-based stereotactic radiosurgery treatment in addition to joined strategies in patients with back uveal melanoma in stage T2/T3, the stereotactic radiosurgery is a successful strategy to treat middle of the road phase of uveal melanoma. At last, one-venture LINAC-based SRS with a solitary portion 35.0 Gy can treat patients with center back uveal melanoma and save the eyeball or be the initial step of consolidated strategies: illumination before endoresection or cyclectomy.

Conflict of interest

None of the authors has conflict of interest with this submission.

Printed form supported by KEGA 023 STU-4/2020, VEGA 1/0395/21, APVV - 17 – 0369.

DOI: http://dx.doi.org/10.5772/intechopen.95321

Author details

Kristina Horkovicova and Alena Furdova*
Department of Ophthalmology, Faculty of Medicine, Comenius University, Bratislava, Slovakia

*Address all correspondence to: alikafurdova@gmail.com; furdova1@uniba.sk

References

[1] Furdova A, Sramka M. Uveal Malignant Melanoma and Stereotactic Radiosurgery: Intraocular Uveal Melanoma and One-Day Session Stereotactic Radiosurgery at Linear Accelerator. Saarbrücken: LAP LAMBERT Academic Publishing; 2014 188 p

[2] Furdova A, Strmen P, Waczulikova I, Chorvath M, Sramka M, Slezak P. One-day session LINAC–based stereotactic radiosurgery of posterior uveal melanoma. European Journal of Ophthalmology. 2012;**22**(2):226-235

[3] Furdová A, Oláh Z. Histologically verified intraocular tumors in the Slovak Republic 1984-1989. Ceská a Slovenská Oftalmologie. 1995 Oct;**51**(5):284-288

[4] Shields JA, Tumors SCLI. An Atlas and Textbook. Philadelphia, Pa: Lippincott Williams & Wilkins; 2008. p. 598

[5] Damato B. Ocular treatment of choroidal melanoma in relation to the prevention of metastatic death - a personal view. Progress in Retinal and Eye Research. 2018 Sep;**66**:187-199

[6] Damato B. Recent developments in ocular oncology. In: Grzybowski A, editor. Current Concepts in Ophthalmology. Springer International Publishing; 2020. pp. 275-293

[7] Damato BE, Singh AD, editors. Clinical Ophthalmic Oncology: Uveal Tumors [Internet]. 3rd ed. Springer International Publishing; 2019 [cited 2020 Mar 19]. Available from: https://www.springer.com/gp/book/9783030178789

[8] Shields CL, Mashayekhi A, Shields JA. By sleight of hand, prognosis determined-even for small choroidal melanoma. JAMA Ophthalmol. 2018 May 1;**136**(5):488-489

[9] Laver NV, McLaughlin ME, Duker JS. Ocular melanoma. Archives of Pathology & Laboratory Medicine. 2010 Dec;**134**(12):1778-1784

[10] Collaborative Ocular Melanoma Study Group. The COMS randomized trial of iodine 125 brachytherapy for choroidal melanoma: V. Twelve-year mortality rates and prognostic factors: COMS report No. 28. Arch Ophthalmol Chic Ill 1960. 2006 Dec;124(12):1684-93.

[11] Collaborative Ocular Melanoma Study Group. Assessment of metastatic disease status at death in 435 patients with large choroidal melanoma in the Collaborative Ocular Melanoma Study (COMS): COMS report no. 15. Arch Ophthalmol Chic Ill 1960. 2001 May;119(5):670-6.

[12] Diener-West M, Reynolds SM, Agugliaro DJ, Caldwell R, Cumming K, Earle JD, et al. Development of metastatic disease after enrollment in the COMS trials for treatment of choroidal melanoma: Collaborative Ocular Melanoma Study Group Report No. 26. Arch Ophthalmol Chic Ill 1960. 2005 Dec;123(12):1639-43.

[13] Honavar SG. Is collaborative ocular melanoma study (COMS) still relevant? Indian Journal of Ophthalmology. 2018;**66**(10):1385-1387

[14] Shields CL, Naseripour M, Cater J, Shields JA, Demirci H, Youseff A, et al. Plaque radiotherapy for large posterior uveal melanomas (> or =8-mm thick) in 354 consecutive patients. Ophthalmology. 2002 Oct;**109**(10):1838-1849

[15] Shields CL, Cater J, Shields JA, Singh AD, Santos MC. Carvalho C. combination of clinical factors predictive of growth of small choroidal

melanocytic tumors. Arch Ophthalmol chic ill 1960. Mar. 2000;**118**(3):360-364

[16] Muller K, Naus N, Nowak PJCM, Schmitz PIM, de Pan C, van Santen CA, et al. Fractionated stereotactic radiotherapy for uveal melanoma, late clinical results. Radiother Oncol J Eur Soc Ther Radiol Oncol. 2012 Feb;**102**(2):219-224

[17] Furdova A, Sramka M, Chorvath M, Kralik G, Furda R, Gregus M. Clinical experience of stereotactic radiosurgery at a linear accelerator for intraocular melanoma. Melanoma Research. 2017 Oct;**27**(5):463-468

[18] Furdova A, Sramka M, Chorvath M, Kralik G, Krasnik V, Krcova I, et al. Stereotactic radiosurgery in intraocular malignant melanoma--retrospective study. Neuro Endocrinology Letters. 2014;**35**(1):28-36

[19] Furdova A, Strmen P, Sramka M. Complications in patients with uveal melanoma after stereotactic radiosurgery and brachytherapy. Bratislavské Lekárske Listy. 2005;**106**(12):401, 16642665-406

[20] Furdova A, Babal P, Kobzova D, Zahorjanova P, Kapitanova K, Sramka M, et al. Uveal melanoma survival rates after single dose stereotactic radiosurgery. Neoplasma. 2018 Nov 15;**65**(6):965-971

[21] Dieckmann K, Georg D, Zehetmayer M, Bogner J, Georgopoulos M, Pötter R. LINAC based stereotactic radiotherapy of uveal melanoma: 4 years clinical experience. Radiotherapy and Oncology. 2003 May;**67**(2):199-206

[22] Dieckmann K, Georg D, Bogner J, Zehetmayer M, Petersch B, Chorvat M, et al. Optimizing LINAC-based stereotactic radiotherapy of uveal melanomas: 7 years' clinical experience. Int J Radiat Oncol • Biol • Phys. 2006 Nov 15;**66**(4):S47-S52

[23] Shields CL, Kaliki S, Furuta M, Fulco E, Alarcon C, Shields JA. American joint committee on cancer classification of posterior uveal melanoma (tumor size category) predicts prognosis in 7731 patients. Ophthalmology. 2013 Oct;**120**(10):2066-2071

[24] Arnett ALH, Reynolds MM, Pulido JS, Parney IF, Laack NN. Gamma knife stereotactic radiosurgery for the treatment of primary and metastatic ocular malignancies. Stereotactic and Functional Neurosurgery. 2017 Nov 4;**95**(6):363-368

[25] Mosci C, Mosci S, Barla A, Squarcia S, Chauvel P, Iborra N. Proton beam radiotherapy of uveal melanoma: Italian patients treated in Nice, France. European Journal of Ophthalmology. 2009 Aug;**19**(4):654-660

[26] Henderson MA, Shirazi H, Lo SS, Mendonca MS, Fakiris AJ, Witt TC, et al. Stereotactic radiosurgery and fractionated stereotactic radiotherapy in the treatment of uveal melanoma. Technology in Cancer Research & Treatment. 2006 Aug;**5**(4):411-419

Chapter 3

Ocular Melanoma

Harika Regani and Santosh G. Honavar

Abstract

Ocular melanoma is the most common malignant tumor in adults after cutaneous melanoma. There is a wide clinical spectrum depending upon the location of the tumor. The various predispositions, risk factors, tumor classification, and treatment modalities are discussed. Choroidal melanoma is the most common type of ocular melanoma. Its management has evolved over the years. The Collaborative Ocular Melanoma Study (COMS) has helped to precisely classify choroidal melanoma and standardize its treatment. The future lies in the genetics which can help prognosticate and provide adjuvant treatment to patients at risk.

Keywords: melanoma, plaque brachytherapy, coms

1. Introduction

The incidence of melanoma continues to rise globally with significant mortality in spite of modern treatment protocols [1]. Ocular melanoma is the most common type of melanoma in adults after the cutaneous melanoma. It constitutes 3.7% of all melanomas [2]. It results due to the abnormal proliferation of the melanocytes in the eye. Based on the location, the ocular melanoma can be broadly classified as follows:

1. Eyelid melanoma
2. Conjunctival melanoma
3. Uveal melanoma
    a. Iris melanoma
    b. Trabecular meshwork melanoma
    c. Iridotrabeculociliary or iridociliary melanoma
    d. Ciliary body melanoma
    e. Choroidal melanoma
    f. Ciliochoroidal melanoma

2. Eyelid melanoma

Eyelid melanoma is relatively and comprises less than 1% of all eyelid cancers. Serial documentation and close monitoring of suspicious lesions play a very important role in early diagnosis. Variable pigmentation, rapid increase in size, change in color, abnormal vascularity, and tendency to bleed are the typical features of eyelid melanoma [3].

3. Conjunctival melanoma

3.1 Epidemiology

The clinical spectrum of melanocytic tumors of the conjunctiva constitutes about 53% of all conjunctival tumors. The reported incidence is two cases per million per year, but the incidence is increasing. It usually occurs at a median age of 62 years and is very rare in children [4, 5].

3.2 Risk factors

1. PAM: 22% (overall: 9%, with atypia: 13%, and without atypia: 0%)

2. Preexisting nevus in 15%

3. De novo 5% [6, 7]

4. Dysplastic nevus syndrome

5. Neurofibromatosis

6. Xeroderma pigmentosum [8]

3.3 Clinical presentation

1. Fleshy, variably pigmented (tan to dark brown) placoid, or modular elevated lesion located on the limbal, bulbar, forniceal, or palpebral conjunctiva. The lesions which are localized, bulbar, thin, and limbal have a good prognosis where as those which are large, diffuse, forniceal, on caruncle and tarsus have poorer prognosis (**Figure 1**).

2. Prominent feeder vessels (conjunctival and scleral)

3. It can develop secondarily in contiguity with an eyelid margin which is called as implantation melanoma [9].

3.4 Treatment

1. A careful dissection of the mass with "no-touch technique," wide excision with frozen section margin control is ideal.

2. Alcohol keratoepitheliectomy for the corneal involvement.

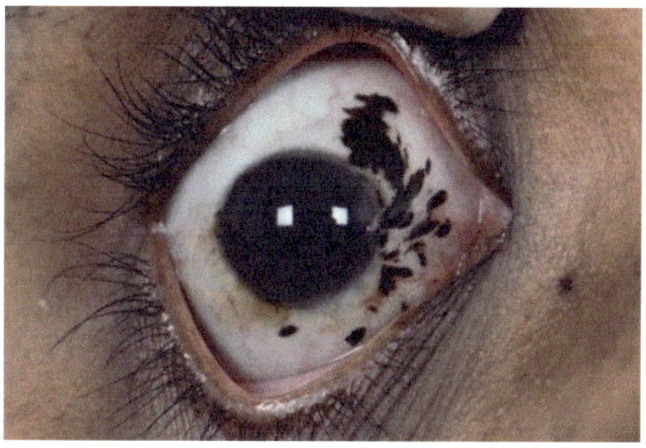

Figure 1.
Conjunctival melanoma.

3. Double freeze thaw cryotherapy of the resection edge and the clinically suspected involved base if it is less than 3 clock hours.

4. Episcleral plaque brachytherapy if base is involved for more than 3 clock hours. Plaque rotation can be customized depending on the tumor extent.

5. Interferon and interleukin-2 in combination can be administered in disseminated melanoma [8].

6. Sentinel lymphangiography is indicated in tumors more than 2 mm and helps in complete removal of the lymph nodes.

3.5 Histopathology

Abnormal proliferation of the melanocytes, spindle, or the epitheloid cells.

3.6 Prognosis

1. Metastasis to ipsilateral facial lymph nodes, brain, lung, skin, bone, and liver are the most common.

2. Multiple recurrences, especially those within the orbit, might require orbital exenteration [4].

3. Intraocular and intraorbital involvement may require modified enucleation and orbital exenteration, respectively.

4. Recurrences after the therapy are 50–70% at 10 years.

5. Overall mortality rate is 25% at 10 years and more than 30% in 15 years [9, 10].

6. The 10 year rate of metastasis is PAM 25%, Nevus 26%, De novo 49% [11]

7. The prognosis can be predicted by the AJCC-TNM staging of conjunctival melanoma (**Table 1**).

8. The factors predictive of metastasis or death are de novo origin, tarsal or forniceal location, nodular mass, and orbital invasion [11].

3.7 Newer innovations

Definition of primary clinical tumor (cT)
TX Primary tumor cannot be assessed
T0 No evidence of primary tumor
T1 Tumor of the bulbar conjunctiva
T1a < 1 quadrant
T1b > 1 but <2 quadrants
T1c > 2 but <3 quadrants
T2 Tumor of nonbulbar conjunctiva (forniceal, palpebral, tarsal, caruncle)
T2a Noncaruncular and < 1 quadrant nonbulbar conjunctiva
T2b Noncaruncular and > 1 quadrant nonbulbar conjunctiva
T2c Caruncular and < 1 quadrant nonbulbar conjunctiva
T2d Caruncular and > 1 quadrant nonbulbar conjunctiva
T3 Tumor of any size with local invasion
T3a Globe
T3b Eyelid
T3c Orbit
T3d Nasolacrimal duct and/or lacrimal sac and/or paranasal sinuses
T4 Tumor of any size with invasion of central nervous system.
Definition of regional lymph nodes (N)
NX Regional lymph nodes cannot be assessed
N0 Regional lymph node metastasis absent
N1 Regional lymph node metastasis present
Definition of distant metastasis (M)
M0 Distant metastasis absent
M1 Distant metastasis present
Definition of primary pathological tumor (pT)
TX Primary tumor cannot be assessed
T0 No evidence or primary tumor
Tis Tumor confined to conjunctival epithelium
T1 Tumor of bulbar conjunctiva
T1a Tumor with <2 mm thickness invasion of substantia propria
T1b Tumor with >2 mm thickness invasion of substantia propria
T2 Tumor of nonbulbar conjunctiva
T2a Tumor with <2 mm thickness invasion of substantia propria
T2b Tumor with >2 mm thickness invasion of substantia propria
T3 Tumor of any size with local invasion
T3a Globe
T3b Eyelid
T3c Orbit
T3d Nasolacrimal duct and/or lacrimal sac and/or paranasal sinuses
T4 Tumor of any size with invasion of central nervous system

Table 1.
AJCC 8th edition classification of conjunctival melanoma.

1. Pembrolizumab—for recurrent conjunctival tumors [12]

2. Nivolumab [13]

4. Uveal melanoma

It is the most common primary intraocular malignancy in adults. The earlier detection and prompt treatment has decreased the morbidity to some extent over the years.

Based on the location, they can be classified into

a. Iris melanoma

b. Trabecular meshwork melanoma

c. Iridotrabeculociliary or iridociliary melanoma

d. Ciliary body melanoma

e. Choroidal melanoma

f. Ciliochoroidal melanoma

The most common differential diagnosis of uveal melanoma is anevus. The following are the key points to differentiate the two (pneumonic: ABCDEF):

1. Age $\leq$ 40 years

2. Blood vessels

3. Clock hours inferiorly

4. Diffuse configuration

5. Ectropion uveae

6. Feathery margin

4.1 Iris melanoma

4.1.1 Epidemiology

Iris melanoma constitutes about 4% of uveal melanomas [14]. The mean age at presentation is 40–47 years. It is very rarely seen in the pediatric age group. Males and females are equally affected. It is most commonly seen in Caucasians (97.8%) [15].

4.1.2 Clinical presentation

Nodular pigmented lesion usually seen in the inferior iris. It is usually associated with tumor seeding in the adjacent iris or trabecular meshwork and secondary glaucoma.

4.1.3 Types

1. Circumscribed

2. Diffuse

4.1.4 Management

1. Observation of clinically suspicious lesions

2. Local resection (iridectomy/iridocyclectomy) for tumors less than 3–4 clock hours

3. Plaque brachytherapy—has up to 87% chance if tumor control after local resection

4. Proton beam therapy

5. Enucleation—for diffuse, recurrent tumors or eyes with intractable glaucoma

4.1.5 Differential diagnosis

1. Primary iris cyst

2. Iris nevus

3. Essential iris atrophy

4. Iris foreign body

5. Peripheral anterior synechiae

6. Iris metastasis

4.1.6 Factors predictive of metastasis

1. Increased age at diagnosis [16, 17]

2. Angle invasion

3. Elevated intraocular pressure

4. Extraocular extension

5. Previous surgical intervention before referral prognosis [14]

Prognosis is better than ciliary body or choroidal melanoma with a 10-year metastasis of 7% as compared to 25% in choroidal melanoma and 34% for ciliary body melanoma.

4.2 Ciliary body melanoma

It is relatively a rare uveal tumor and is reported in one of 10 cases of all intraocular melanomas [18, 19].

4.2.1 Clinical presentation

1. Diminution of vision due to astigmatism or lens dislocation

2. Painless visual field loss or pain due to acute glaucoma

3. Episcleral sentinel vessels

4. Unexplained relatively low intraocular pressure

Management options include local resection, plaque brachytherapy, proton beam radiation, and enucleation.

4.2.2 Histopathological types (callender classification)

1. Spindle A and B type melanoma—best prognosis
2. Mixed cell melanoma
3. Epitheloid cell melanoma—poor prognosis
4. Necrotic melanoma—poor prognosis

4.2.3 Metastasis

Hematogenous metastasis is faster in ciliary body melanoma as a result of continuous contractions of the ciliary muscle and rich vascularization.

T Category and criteria
T1—Tumor limited to the iris T1a—Tumor limited to the iris, not more than 3 clock hours in size T1b—Tumor limited to the iris, more than 3 clock hours in size T1c—Tumor limited to the iris with secondary glaucoma T2—Tumor confluent with or extending into the ciliary body, choroid, or both T2a—Tumor confluent with or extending into the ciliary body, without secondary glaucoma T2b—Tumor confluent with or extending into the ciliary body and choroid, without secondary glaucoma T2c—Tumor confluent with or extending into the ciliary body, choroid, or both with secondary glaucoma
T3—Tumor confluent with or extending into the ciliary body, choroid, or both, with scleral extension
T4—Tumor with extrascleral extension T4a—Tumor with extrascleral extension $\leq$5 mm in largest diameter T4b Tumor with extrascleral extension >5 mm in largest diameter
G Category and criteria
GX—Grade cannot be assessed G1—Spindle cell melanoma (>90% spindle cells) G2—Mixed cell melanoma (>10% epitheloid cells and < 90% spindle cells) G3—Epitheloid cell melanoma (>90% epitheloid cells)
N Category and criteria
N1—Regional lymph node metastasis or discrete tumor deposits in the orbit N1a—Metastasis in one or more regional lymph node(s) N1b—No regional lymph nodes are positive, but there are discrete tumor deposits in the orbit that are not contiguous to the eye
M Category and criteria
M0—No distant metastasis by clinical classification M1—Distant metastasis M1a—Largest diameter of the largest metastasis $\leq$3 cm M1b—Largest diameter of the largest metastasis 3.1–8 cm M1c—Largest diameter of the largest metastasis $\geq$8.1 cm

Table 2.
AJCC 8th edition classification of iris melanoma [20].

Clinical	Macroscopic	Microscopic
Local/general signs	Size of the tumor	Epitheloid and necrotic cellular patterns
Local extension	<11 mm—small	Necrosis
Presence of metastasis	11–15 mm—medium	Intense pigmentation
Age of the patient	>15 mm—large	Melanophagic, lymphocytic infiltrate
Dysplastic nevi		

Table 3.
The prognostic factors for ciliary body melanoma.

Host factors	Environment factors
Light colored eyes	Intermittent ultraviolet exposure to arc welding
Fair skinned	Chronic UV exposure
	Occupational sunlight exposure

Table 4.
Predisposing factors.

4.2.4 Prognosis

The prognostic factors are listed in **Table 3**.

4.3 Choroidal melanoma

Choroidal melanoma is the most common uveal melanoma and constitutes about 90% of all uveal melanomas. This is usually seen in an elderly age group at around 60 years and there is no gross gender predilection. It is seen predominantly in Caucasians (98%), as compared to other races. It has a pronounced tendency to metastasize resulting in high mortality [21]. Predisposing factors are listed in **Table 4**.

4.3.1 Clinical presentation

It can be incidentally detected in asymptomatic patients on routine ocular examination. Most of the patients, however, manifest with diminution of vision, floaters, photopsia, visual field loss, or pain due to impingement of posterior ciliary nerve or angle closure glaucoma. It can metastasize to liver (89%), lung (29%), and bone (17%). Median survival after metastasis is 6–12 months [22]. Males have a poor prognosis than females. The lower metastatic rate in females can be explained due to the inhibitory action of estrogen on the growth of micrometastases within the liver [23, 24].

4.3.2 Classification

Choroidal melanoma can be broadly classified into diffuse (**Figure 2**) and circumscribed (**Figure 3**). The circumscribed variant can either be dome-shaped (75%) or mushroom-shaped (20%). Diffuse choroidal melanoma is seen in 3–17% cases and has a substantial risk of metastasis despite its flat appearance. The poor prognostic factors include delayed diagnosis, greater proportion of epitheloid cells, and a tendency for extraocular extension [25].

AJCC Classification has already been mentioned under the section of iris melanoma (**Table 2**).

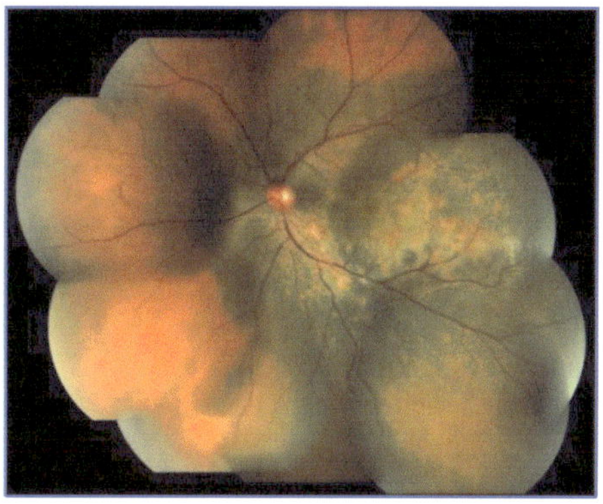

Figure 2.
Diffuse choroidal melanoma.

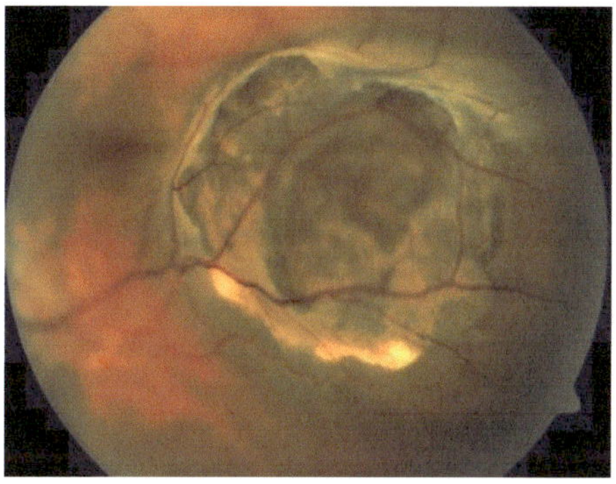

Figure 3.
Circumscribed choroidal melanoma.

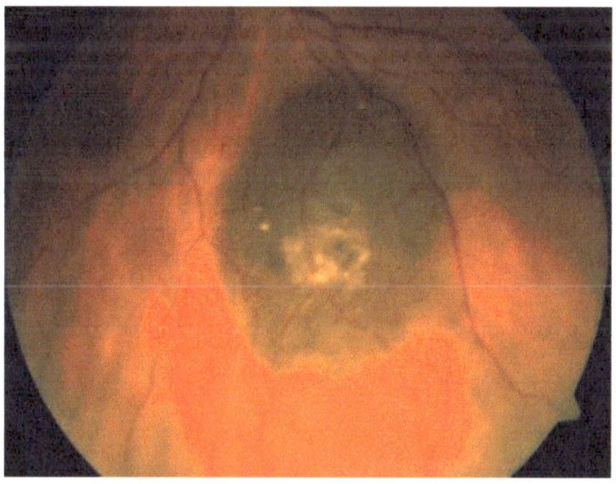

Figure 4.
Choroidal nevus.

The most common precursor lesion for choroidal melanoma is the preexisting choroidal nevus (**Figure 4**), followed by oculodermal melanocytosis.

The following are used to differentiate a choroidal nevus from a melanoma (pneumonic: to find small ocular melanoma using helpful hints daily):

1. Thickness > 2 mm

2. Fluid

3. Symptoms

4. Orange pigmentation

5. Margin <3 mm to disk

6. Ultrasound hollow

7. Absent halo

8. Absent grusen

4.3.3 Investigations

4.3.3.1. Ultrasonography

It has 95% accuracy and is useful to estimate tumor size for periodic observation and to evaluate for extraocular extension.

The characteristic features on A-scan are:

1. Initial prominent spike

2. Low to medium internal reflectivity with diminishing amplitude

3. Fine oscillation of internal spiking pattern (vascular pulsations)

The characteristic features on B-scan are:

1. Low to medium internal reflectivity

2. Choroidal excavation

3. Shadowing of subadjacent soft tissue

4. Internal vascularity

5. Acoustic hallowing

4.3.3.2. Autofloroscence

Hyperautofluorescence of orange-colored lipofuscin pigment.

4.3.3.3. Fundus fluorescein angiography

Small melanoma: Hypofluorescence (blocked fluorescence)

Large melanoma: Patchy pattern of early hypofluorescence and hyperfluorescence followed by late intense staining. Double circulation—internal vascularity

4.3.3.4. Ultrasound biomicroscopy

It helps to differentiate anterior tumors from those of ciliary body origin. Although the tumor margins and extent is well delineated by UBM, the resolution of internal tumor details is limited.

4.3.3.5. Optical coherence tomography

Dome-shaped choroidal mass with overlying outer retinal thickening and subretinal fluid.

Optical coherence tomography angiography shows reduced capillary density in the affected eye.

4.3.3.6. Magnetic resonance imaging

Pigmented melanomas can be seen as T1 Hyperdense and T2 hypodense intraocular masses.

4.3.3.7. Fine needle aspiration cytology

Although reliable, it is technically challenging and requires expertise.

4.3.4 Management

The most common treatment modality is the episceral plaque brachytherapy. Plaque brachytherapy is suitable for tumors up to 16 mm in diameter and up to 6 mm thickness with Ruthenium-106 and up to 8 mm thickness with Iodine-125. The dose to the tumor apex should be 10,000 cGy and almost up to 90% tumor control can be achieved. Enucleation is an option for tumors beyond the scope of plaque brachytherapy. Orbital exenteration might be required in tumors with orbital invasion. The proton beam irradiation has a higher chance of eye salvage but the availability and affordability are the considerable limitations. The other treatment modalities include laser photocoagulation, transpupillary thermotherapy, chemotherapy, and immunotherapy.

The various newer treatment modalities under evaluation are:

1. Chemotherapy with dacarbazine+interferon alpha, cisplatin, tamoxifen +sunitinib, and fotemustine.

2. Targeted therapy with crizotinib, sunitinib, and valproic acid.

3. Immunotherapy with Ipilimumab with nivolumab.

4.3.5 Histopathology

Modified Callenders's classification describes various patterns on histopathology.

1. Spindle cell nevi

2. Spindle cell melanoma

3. Necrotic melanoma

4. Epitheloid cell melanoma

5. Mixed cell melanoma

Clinical features	Histopathologic features	Cytogenetic features	Transcriptomic feature
Older age at presentation	Epithelioid cytology	Chromosome 3 loss (monosomy 3)	Gene expression profile class 2
Male gender	High mitotic activity/PC-10/Ki-67	Chromosome 8q gain or 8p loss	
Larger tumor basal diameter	High values of mean diameter of 10 largest nucleoli	Chromosome 1p loss	
Thicker tumor	High microvascular density	Chromosome 6q loss	
Ciliary body tumor location	Microvascular loops and patterns	Chromosome 9q loss	
Diffuse tumor configuration	Tumor-infiltrating lymphocytes, macrophages	BAP1 loss	
Association with ocular/oculodermal melanocytosis	Loss of nuclear immunostaining for BAP1		
Extraocular tumor extension	High expression of insulin-like growth factor 1 receptor		
Advanced AJCC category and staging	High expression of HLA class I and II		

Table 5.
The poor prognostic factors include [26].

The epitheloid cell and the mixed cell melanoma have the poorest prognosis among all the subtypes (**Table 5**). Immunohistochemical markers characteristic of choroidal melanoma are S-100, HMB-45.

4.3.6 Metastasis

The risk factors for metastasis include (**Table 7**):

1. Thickness > 2 mm

2. Symptoms

3. Margin <3 mm to disk

4. Documented growth

The presence of four risk factors has a metastatic rate of 20% but the absence of risk factors has only <1% risk of systemic metastasis. Also, each millimeter increase in thickness adds 5% risk for metastasis at 10 years and a hazard ratio of 1.08 [27]. Doubling time of untreated metastases ranged from 34 to 220 days (median, 63 days). The metastasis from tumors as small as 3 × 3 × 1.5 mm has been noted in a study [28]. Based on the estimated growth rates, a rational follow-up interval to detect metastatic uveal melanoma would be 4–6 months. Primary uveal melanomas that develop clinically detectable metastasis after conservative therapy may have micrometastasized several years before treatment.

Damato's classification of metastasis [26]:

1. Metastasizing melanomas, which have already metastasized by the time of ocular treatment even though the metastases may not be detectable.

2. Pre-metastasizing melanomas, which develop metastatic capability and disseminate if treatment is delayed.

3. Non-metastasizing melanomas, which do not metastasize even if never treated.

4.3.7 Colloborative ocular melanoma study

This is the largest study ever to be performed in Ocular oncology with 43 participating centers and more than 2000 patients [29, 30].

Objectives of the study:

1. To evaluate the therapeutic interventions for patients with choroidal melanoma

2. To determine which of the two, enucleation or brachytherapy prolongs the lifetime of an individual, and if both have a similar survival, then which offers the longer cancer-free survival and better prognosis for vision.

Inclusion and exclusion criteria:

- Primary choroidal melanoma in one eye
- Less than 50% involvement of ciliary body
- Age 21 years or older
- Ability to give informed consent
- Ability to return for treatment and scheduled follow-up
- No primary cancer (except noninvasive nonmelanotic skin cancer/CIS cervix)
- No coexisting disease threatening survival (5 years or longer)
- No metastatic melanoma
- No contraindication for surgery/RT
- No previous FNAB
- No previous treatment
- No extrascleral extension of 2 mm or more
- No diffuse, ring or multifocal tumor
- No iris/angle involvement
- No use of immunosuppressive therapy that cannot be discontinued

Outcome measures:

1. Primary outcome: Time to death from all-cause mortality

2. Secondary outcome: Metastasis-free survival, cancer-free survival, and years of useful vision

Trial design and treatment groups:

1. Small <3 (1.5–2.4) mm, 5 mm (observational group)

2. Medium 3–8 (2.5–10) mm, 16 mm (randomized group)

3. Large >8 (10 mm), >16 mm (randomized group)

Results:

1. Pre-enucleation EBRT for large melanoma has no advantage over enucleation group. Five-year Kaplan–Meier estimates for survival were 57% for the enucleation group and 62% for the pre enucleation radiation group.

2. Enucleation versus brachytherapy for medium melanoma were comparable. The cumulative all-cause mortality at 12 years was 43% for patient in the plaque radiotherapy group versus 41% for those in enucleation group.

3. The small tumor trial showed that small choroidal melanomas managed by observation showed tumor growth in 21% by 2 years and 31% by 5 years. Observation for small melanoma is not acceptable now and is treated appropriately.

4.3.8 Genetic markers

The mitogen-activated protein kinase (MAPK) pathway is one of the main regulatory pathways involved in choroidal melanoma development, particularly through mutations in BRAF, NRAS, and KIT. Choroidal melanoma with BRAF mutation is common in younger patients and the ones associated with preexisting nevi. KIT mutations are the least common choroidal melanoma mutation in MAPK pathway. NRAS mutation is very rare in choroidal melanoma [21–33]. Disomy 3 and chromosome 6p gain are associated with a good prognosis.

Chromosome 3 loss, 8q gain, 1p loss and 6q loss = Class 1 associated with poor prognosis.

Based on gene expression prolifes (GEP), uveal melanoma is now classified into three prognostic categories for metastasis (**Table 6**).

The GEPs are playing a major role at present in prognosticating the risk of metastasis. The tumor as such is constantly evolving at the genetic and molecular level which is described as intratumoral genetic heterogeneity. The term cresendo malignancy is described which explains the transformation of a small tumor which is slow growing over years but acquires Class 2 genetic changes over time (**Table 6**).

		Systemic metastasis at 5 years
Class 1A	Low risk	2%
Class 1B	Intermediate risk	21%
Class 2	High risk	72%

Table 6.
Prognostic categories for metastasis.

Tumor size	Monosomy 3	If M3, metastasis by 3 years
Small 0–3 mm	23%	0%
Med 3–8 mm	35%	24%
Large >8 mm	>50%	58%

Table 7.
Metastasis depends on several factors: Size, markers-BAPI, and genetics [34].

4.3.9 Follow-up

A periodic follow-up with systemic investigations is mandatory in view of high metastatic rates of choroidal melanoma. An annual PET-CT scan is ideal, however, the monitoring of the liver function tests, ultrasonography of the abdomen and the chest X-Ray are reasonably good.

5. Conclusion

Ocular melanoma is being effectively managed currently. A protocol-based management of the patient can lead to good local tumor control and careful systemic monitoring can decrease the morbidity and mortality to a great extent. The ongoing research in genetics will probably help us understand and prognosticate ocular melanoma in a better way.

Acknowledgements

The authors acknowledge this chapter to their patients.

Conflict of interest

The authors declare no conflict of interest.

Author details

Harika Regani* and Santosh G. Honavar
Centre for Sight Superspeciality Eye Hospital, Hyderabad, India

*Address all correspondence to: harikaregani@gmail.com

References

[1] GLOBOCAN 2012 v1.0, Cancer Incidence and Mortality Worldwide: IARC Cancer Base No. 11 [Internet]. 2013 [Cited: April 6, 2017]. Available from: http://globocan.iarc.fr. [Accessed: 26 July 2020]

[2] McLaughlin CC, Wu XC, Jemal A, Martin HJ, Ro-Che LM, Chen VW. Incidence of noncutaneous melanomas in the U.S. Cancer. 2005;**103**:1000-1007

[3] Paul TF. Malignant Melanoma of the Eyelid. New York: Eye Cancer Centre; Available from: Eyecancer.com

[4] Shields CL, Shields JA, Gunduz K, et al. Conjunctival melanoma: risk factors for recurrence, exenteration, metastasis, and death in 150 consecutive patients. Arch Ophthalmol. 2000;**118**(11):1497-1507

[5] Stremnel I, Kroll P. Conjunctival malignant melanoma in children. Journal of Ophthalmology. 1999;**213**: 129-132

[6] Shields CL, Shields JA. Tumors of the conjunctiva and cornes. Survey of Ophthalmology. 2004;**49**:3-24

[7] Shields JA, Eyelid SCL. Conjunctival and Orbital Tumors. An Atlas and Textbook. 2nd ed. Philadelphia, PA: Lippincott Williams and Wilkins; 2008. pp. 250-445

[8] Honavar SG, Manjandavida FP. Tumors of the ocular surface. A review. Indian Journal of Ophthalmology. 2015; **63**:187-203

[9] Giblin ME, Shields JA, Shields CL, Eagle RC Jr. Primary eyelid malignant melanoma associated with primary conjunctival malignant melanoma. Australian and New Zealand Journal of Ophthalmology. 1988;**16**:127-131

[10] Shields CL, Demirci H, Karatza E, Shields JA. Clinical survey of 1643 melanocytic and nonmelanocytic conjunctival tumors. Ophthalmology. 2004;**111**:1747-1754

[11] Shields CL, Markowitz JS, Belinsky I, et al. Conjunctival melanoma: Outcomes based on tumor origin in 382 consecutive cases. Ophthalmology. 2011;**118**(2): 389-395.e952. DOI: 10.1016/j.ophtha.2010.06.021

[12] Kini A, Fu R, Compton C, Miller DM, Ramasubramanian A. Pembrolizumab for recurrent conjunctival melanoma. JAMA Ophthalmology. 2017;**135**(8):891-892. DOI: 10.1001/jamaophthalmol.2017.2279

[13] Sagiv O, Thakar SD, Kandl TJ, et al. Immunotherapy with programmed cell death 1 inhibitors for 5 patients with conjunctival melanoma. JAMA Ophthalmology. 2018;**136**(11): 1236-1241. DOI: 10.1001/jamaophthalmol.2018.3488

[14] Shields CL, Kaliki S, Furuta M, et al. Clinical spectrum and prognosis of uveal melanoma based on age at presentation in 8,033 cases. Retina. 2012;**32**(7): 1363-1372

[15] McLaughlin JP, Fung AT, Shields JA, Shields CL. Iris melanoma in children: Current approach to management. Oman Journal of Ophthalmology. 2013; **6**(1):53-55

[16] Shields CL, Kaliki S, Shah SU, Luo W, Furuta M, Shields JA. Iris melanoma: Features and prognosis in 317 children and adults. Journal of AAPOS. 2012;**16**(1):6-10. 7

[17] Shields CL, Shields JA, Materin M, Gershenbaum E, Singh AD, Smith A. Iris melanoma: Risk factors for metastasis in 169 consecutive patients. Ophthalmology. 2001;**108**(1): 172-178

[18] Oittinen HA-L, O'Shaughnessy M, Cullinane AB, et al. Malignant melanoma of the ciliary body presenting as extraocular metastasis in the temporalis muscle. Journal of Clinical Pathology. 2007;**60**:834-835

[19] Costache M et al. Ciliary body melanoma—A particularly rare type of ocular tumor. Case report and general considerations. Maedica. 2013;**8**(4): 360-364

[20] Updated classification for primary iris melanoma [Internet]. 2017. Available from: https://retinatoday.com/articles [Accessed: 26 July 2020]

[21] Kalki S, Shields CL, Shields JA. Uveal melanoma: Estimating prognosis. Indian Journal of Ophthalmology. 2015; **63**:93-102

[22] Diener-West M, Reynolds SM, Agugliaro DJ, Caldwell R, Cumming K, Earle JD, et al. Development of metastatic disease after enrollment in the COMS trials for treatment of choroidal melanoma: Collaborative Ocular Melanoma Study Group Report No 26. Archives of Ophthalmology. 2005;**123**:1639-1643

[23] Zloto O, Pe'er J, Frenkel S. Gender differences in clinical presentation and prognosis of uveal melanoma. Investigative Ophthalmology & Visual Science. 2013;**54**:652-656

[24] Rietschel P, Panageas KS, Hanlon C, Patel A, Abramson DH, Chapman PB. Variates of survival in metastatic uveal melanoma. Journal of Clinical Oncology. 2005;**23**:8076-8080

[25] Shields CL, Kaliki S, Furuta M, Shields JA. Diffuse versus nondiffuse small (=3 MM thickness) choroidal melanoma: Comparative analysis in 1,751 cases. The 2012 F. Phinizy Calhoun lecture. Retina. 2013;**33**:1763-1776

[26] Damato B. Does ocular treatment of uveal melanoma influence survival? British Journal of Cancer. 2010;**103**: 285-290

[27] Shields CL, Furuta M, Thangappan A, et al. Metastasis of uveal melanoma millimeter-by-millimeter in 8033 consecutive eyes. Archives of Ophthalmology. 2009;**127**(8): 989-998. DOI: 10.1001/archophthalmol.2009.208

[28] Eskelin S, Pyrhonen S, Summanen P, Hahka-Kemppinen M, Kivela T. Tumor doubling times in metastatic malignant melanoma of the uvea: Tumor progression before and after treatment. Ophthalmology. 2000; **107**(8):1443-1449. DOI: 10.1016/s0161-6420(00)00182-2

[29] The Collaborative Ocular Melanoma Study (COMS) randomized trial of pre-enucleation radiation of large choroidal melanoma, II: Initial mortality findings. COMS report no. 10. American Journal of Ophthalmology. 1998;**125**:779-796

[30] Hawkins BS, Collaborative Ocular Melanoma Study Group. The Collaborative Ocular Melanoma Study (COMS) randomized trial of pre-enucleation radiation of large choroidal melanoma: IV. Ten-year mortality findings and prognostic factors. COMS report number 24. American Journal of Ophthalmology. 2004;**138**:936-951

[31] Spendlove HE, Damato BE, Humphreys J, Barker KT, Hiscott PS, Houlston RS. BRAF mutations are detectable in conjunctival but not uveal melanomas. Melanoma Research. 2004;**14**(6):449-452. [PubMed: 15577314]

[32] Griewank KG, Westekemper H, Murali R, et al. Conjunctival melanomas harbor BRAF and NRAS mutations and copy number changes similar to cutaneous and mucosal melanomas. Clinical Cancer Research: An Official Journal of the American Association for

Cancer Research. 2013;**19**(12): 3143-3152. [PubMed: 23633454]

[33] Beadling C, Jacobson-Dunlop E, Hodi FS, et al. KIT gene mutations and copy number in melanoma subtypes. Clinical Cancer Research: An Official Journal of the American Association for Cancer Research. 2008;**14**(21): 6821-6828

[34] Shields CL, Ganguly A, Bianciotto CG, Turaka K, Tavallali A, Shields JA. Prognosis of uveal melanoma in 500 cases using genetic testing of fine-needle aspiration biopsy specimens. Ophthalmology. 2011;**118**(2):396-401. DOI: 10.1016/j.ophtha.2010.05.023

Chapter 4

Anorectal Melanoma

Rahul Gupta, Nalini Bansal, Houssem Ammar and Jyoti Gupta

Abstract

Malignant melanoma is an aggressive disease. The anorectal region is the most common site of primary gastrointestinal malignant melanoma. Due to its low incidence, the diagnosis is often delayed. The most characteristic clinical feature of this tumor is its brown-black appearance due to the melanin pigment. However, the pigmentation may be absent in up to 20% cases. Timely diagnosis and treatment are crucial for achieving good long-term outcomes. Surgical excision remains the treatment of choice for localized disease. However, the extent of surgery has been a matter of debate. Anorectal melanoma is a highly malignant disease, and more than 50% cases have metastasis at the time of diagnosis. Targeted therapies especially immune check point inhibitors have brought about a paradigm shift in the management of cutaneous melanoma. They are being increasingly used for mucosal melanomas, and their role in anorectal melanoma is being investigated in various clinical trials.

Keywords: malignant melanoma, anus, rectum, mucosal, check point inhibitors

1. Introduction

Anorectal melanoma (AM) is a rare type of anorectal malignancy. It accounts for about 1% of all anal cancers [1]. Due to its rarity, it is often misdiagnosed as hemorrhoids, rectal adenocarcinoma and polyps. Its early diagnosis and treatment are important to improve the prognosis as it is an aggressive disease with high malignant potential. There are no standard guidelines for the diagnosis, staging and treatment of AM. In this chapter, we have discussed the epidemiological, pathogenesis, clinical manifestations, treatment and prognosis of AM.

2. Epidemiology

Mucosal melanoma (MM) accounts for 1–2% of all melanomas with incidence of 2–2.6 cases per million people/year [2]. The most common sites of MM are head and neck followed by anorectal region [3]. AM is the most common type of gastrointestinal melanoma and the third most common type of melanoma [3]. AM accounts for 16.5% cases of mucosal melanomas [4]. The annual incidence rate of AM is 0.259 in males and 0.407 in females according to Surveillance, Epidemiology, and End Results (SEER) analysis and, the incidence has been steadily increasing over the years [5, 6]. However, the exact reasons for rising incidence are poorly understood. The prevalence of AM is 1.6 to 2.3 times higher in females than males and two times higher in Caucasians than African Americans [7, 8].

3. Pathogenesis and genetics

Melanocytes are derived from the neural crest cells. They migrate to the cutis and mucocutaneous junctions during the embryonal life. The chief function of melanocytes is their antioxidant activity, which helps to counteract the free radicals generated by the ultraviolet rays. Additionally, they contribute to the regional immune response [9, 10]. It has been postulated that the malignant transformation of melanocytes occurs due to oxidative stress and/or immunosuppression [9]. Other theories on AM suggest that they may be derived from Schwann cells of autonomic nervous system or the cells of the amine-precursor uptake and decarboxylation (APUD) system of the gastrointestinal tract [11]. Ultraviolet rays play a central role in the development of cutaneous melanoma (CM) unlike mucosal melanoma (MM). Hence, other pathways are involved in the development of MM which are poorly understood.

MM have different mutation profile compared to cutaneous melanomas [12]. BRAF mutations are infrequent, with an increased rate of c-KIT overexpression [13]. The incidence of BRAF, NRAS and c-KIT mutations are 5–16%, 14–18% and 11–15% respectively [14–16]. The mutation profiles of mucosal melanomas indicate that they have potential sensitivity to CDK4/6 and MEK inhibitors [16]. A study by Newell et al. have identified various mutational signatures in mucosal melanomas [16]. They found that mutations for melanoma in facial sites are different from that found in lower body sites. For example, SF3B1 hotspot mutations are common in AM and vulvovaginal melanomas, unlike other sites. Another study by Donizy et al. found that high poly (ADP-ribose) polymerase 1 (PARP-1) expression alone and along with high indoleamine 2,3-dioxygenase 1 (IDO-1) expression in mucosal melanomas was associated with worse overall and disease-specific survival [17]. Some studies have speculated that some viruses such as human papilloma virus (HPV) and human herpes virus (HHV-8) could be involved in the development of primary MM [11]. However, HPV DNA and HHV-8 DNA could not be detected in cases with AM [18, 19].

4. Clinical features

4.1 Clinical signs and symptoms

The clinical features of AM mimic that of benign anorectal disorders leading to delay in diagnosis. The main clinical symptoms include bleeding per rectum, perianal pain, pruritus ani, tenesmus, perianal mass, inguinal mass (**Figure 1**). It is more frequent in females than males (1.7:1). It is most frequently observed in 6th and 7th decade of life [5]. The most important aspect of clinical diagnosis is a careful perianal and per-rectal examination. AM appears as an ulcerated or nodular lesion with an irregular surface showing brown or black pigmentation (**Figure 1**). Moreover, these are vascular lesions which bleed on touching. Frequently, in about 20% cases, the pigmentation may be absent. In small lesions, a high index of suspicion is required for timely diagnosis due its appearance similar to hemorrhoids. Hence, whenever in doubt, incisional or excisional biopsy should be performed for histopathological examination to diagnose AM. Another important clinical finding in cases of AM is the presence of inguinal lymphadenopathy. Inguinal lymph nodal metastases are usually seen in cases of anal melanoma. In cases with inguinal lymphadenopathy, fine needle aspiration and cytological examination for the enlarged lymph nodes can help in making the diagnosis.

Serum markers can aid in the diagnosis of AM. However, they are elevated in advanced cases of melanoma and often used as an adjunct to the other investigations for diagnosis. Lactate dehydrogenase (LDH) is a commonly used marker

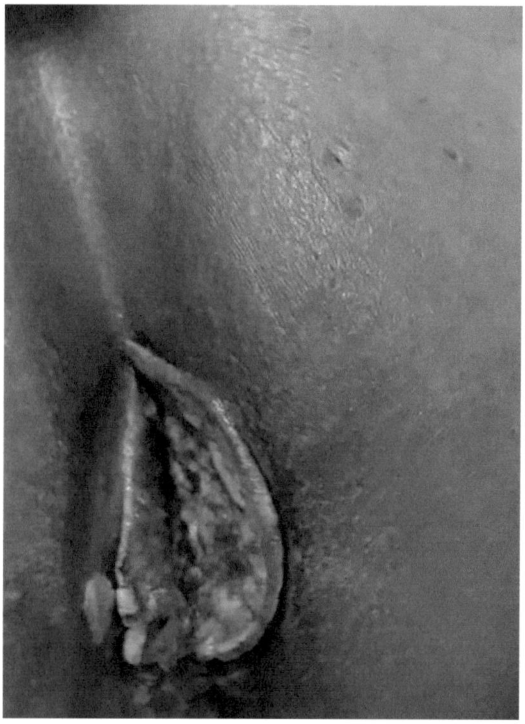

Figure 1.
Perianal examination showing the ulcerated mass in a patient with locally advanced anorectal melanoma.

for the detection of distant metastases in patients with melanoma [20]. Other markers include S-100B, melanoma inhibitor activity (MIA) protein, enolase and YKL-40 [21–24]. Elevated levels of these markers have been associated with a poor prognosis.

4.2 Radiological studies

The main role of radiological investigations is to determine the extent of the disease. Chest radiograph can detect obvious pulmonary metastases while abdominal ultrasound can detect liver metastasis [25]. Computed tomography (CT) is helpful in accurate staging of the disease (**Figure 2**). On CT, the liver lesions show late arterial enhancement and hypoattenuation of liver parenchyma in the portal venous phase [26]. The pulmonary metastases on CT chest appear as multiple end-arterial nodules with tree-in-bud appearance [25]. Magnetic resonance imaging (MRI) is a good imaging modality for accurate assessment of the local invasion of the tumor

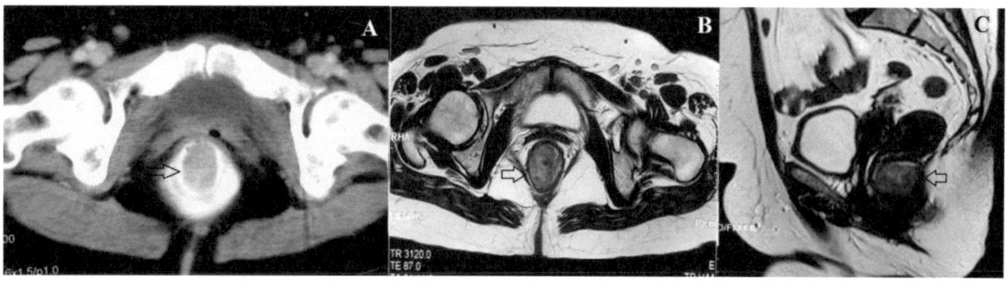

Figure 2.
Anorectal melanoma appeared as a heterogeneously enhancing polypoidal mass (arrow) on contrast enhanced CT (A) and MRI (B, C).

as well as for the detection of metastatic lesions in the liver (**Figure 2**) [27]. PETCT is the recommended imaging for the staging and response assessment of metastatic melanoma [20]. Melanoma cells have higher FDG avidity compared to normal tissues due to high metabolic rate [20].

4.3 Endoscopic studies

For deeply located AM, especially rectal melanoma, endoscopy is very useful to visualize the lesions and take biopsies for histological examination. On endoscopy, the lesions appear as black or brownish plaques, ulcers or polyps due to the melanin pigment. The accuracy of endoscopic biopsy ranges from 50 to 100% [28]. The accuracy is low for lesions with atypical endoscopic characteristics. Endoscopic ultrasound is helpful in determining the depth of the lesions especially the extent of anal sphincter involvement and to look for perirectal lymphadenopathy. The lesions appear hypoechoic with uneven internal echoes [28].

5. Histopathology

As none of the clinical features are unique to AM, histological examination of the suspected lesions should be performed for the definitive diagnosis of AM. The main cytological features of AM are highly cellular smear, presence of binucleated or multinucleated cells, and cytoplasmic melanin pigment. However, melanin pigment is found in only about 27% cases [29].

On gross examination, the lesion appears as polypoidal or ulcerated lesion with or without brown-black pigmentation (**Figure 3**). The histological description includes cell type, degree of melanin pigmentation and mitotic index (Ki-67) [20]. Typically, AM consists of spindle-shaped (**Figure 4**) or epitheloid cells with high nuclear pleomorphism and presence of cytoplasmic melanin granules (**Figure 5**) [30]. About 20% cases are truly amelanotic on histology [31]. Four subtypes of AM based on histology are epitheloid, spindle cell, lymphoma-like and pleomorphic [32]. In the absence of melanin pigments, the tumor morphology can mimic lymphoma and gastrointestinal stromal tumors. Immunohistochemistry helps in differentiate AM from other tumors. Melanoma antigens such as S-100, HMB-45 and vimentin are positive in 78, 94 and 100% cases (**Figure 6**) [31]. The characteristic

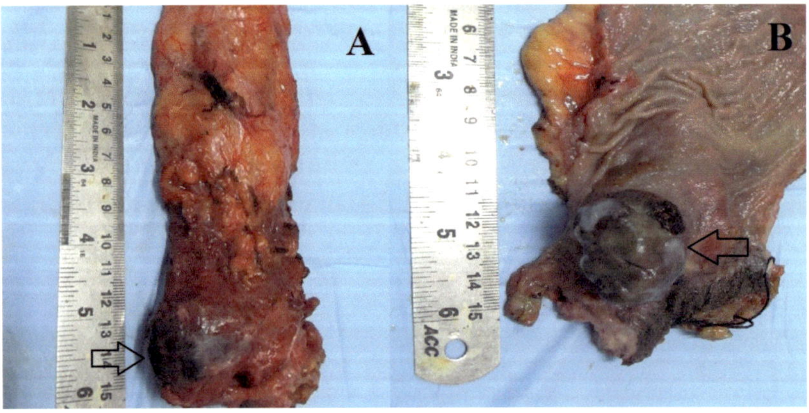

Figure 3.
Gross examination of the specimen after abdominoperineal resection showing the pigmented polypoidal hard growth (arrow) of about 3 cm reaching up to the outer surface (A) and involving the anorectal junction (B).

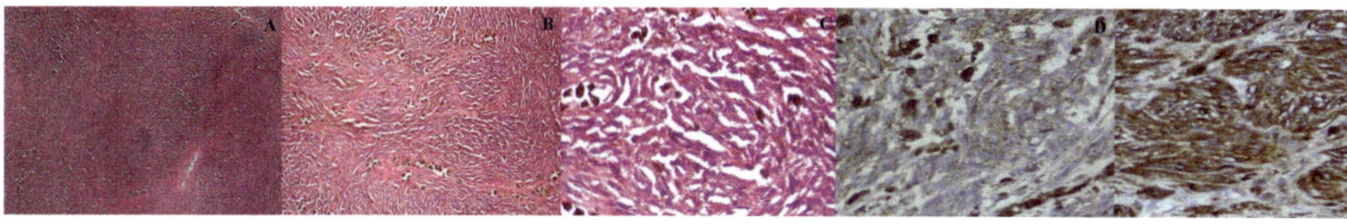

Figure 4.
Histological examination of anorectal melanoma showing the diffuse infiltration of the tissue by spindle-shaped cells with dense eosinophilic cytoplasm and pleomorphic nuclei: (A) H&E x10, (B) H&E x 20, and (C) H&E x 40. Immunohistochemical analysis revealed positive staining with c-KIT (D) and Melan A (E).

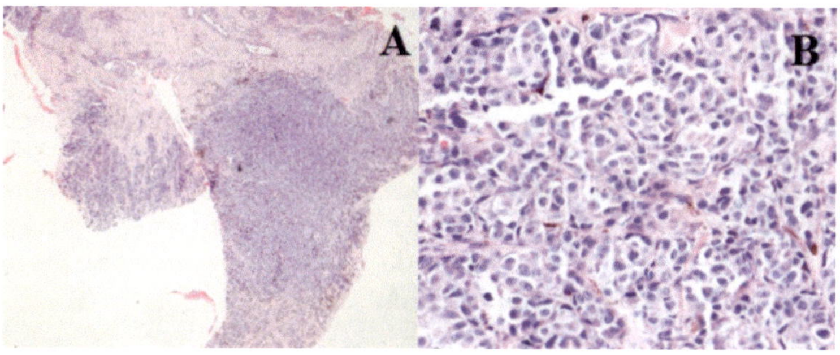

Figure 5.
Microscopic examination of the tumor showing diffuse infiltration of the anorectal region by large epitheloid cells with vesicular and prominent nuclei (A) H&E x 10 and (B) H&E x 40.

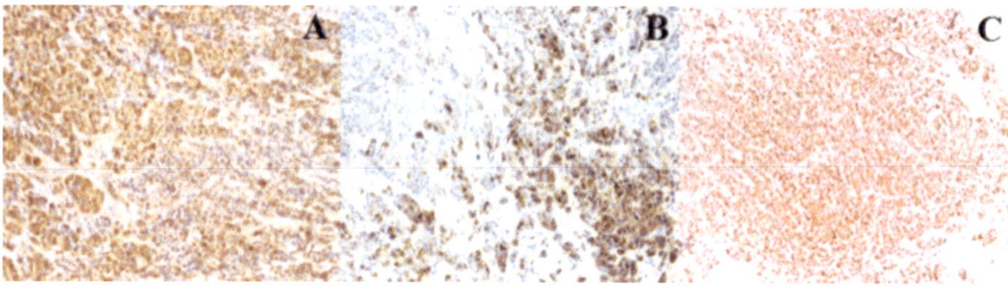

Figure 6.
Immunohistochemical analysis of the anorectal melanoma showing positivity for HMB 45 (A), Melan A (B) and SOX 10 (C).

marker of gastrointestinal stromal tumor, c-Kit is positive in about three-fourth cases of AM (**Figure 4**) [32]. In some cases, the tumor cells may show positivity for CEA, CD30 and CD68 similar to colorectal adenocarcinoma and other tumors [33]. Hence, a panel of markers should be tested to confirm the diagnosis of AM in doubtful cases. Some unique markers for melanoma with high specificity and low sensitivity include Melanin A, Mart-1 antibodies [20]. Interestingly, Ki-67 and proliferating cell nuclear antigen (PCNA) immunostains have been found to predict survival in patients with AM [31].

Tumor-infiltrating lymphocytes (TILs) provide a reflection of the tumor microenvironment. Presence of TILs in high concentration is associated with high programmed cell death protein 1 (PD-1) [34]. High PD-1 expression indicates better prognosis for patients with AM due to good response to targeted therapies. TILs can be seen on hematoxylin and eosin stains and also with immunohistochemistry. The majority of these TILs are CD8-positive cells. In a study of 43 AM patients, TILs were present in 55% cases [35].

6. Diagnosis and staging

As CM and MM are known for early hematogenous spread, secondary gastrointestinal melanomas are not rare. Hence, for differentiation between primary and secondary melanoma, the following criteria must be satisfied: absence of melanoma at any other cutaneous or mucosal sites confirmed by thorough clinical including genital, oropharyngeal, ophthalmological and endoscopic examination; no past history of melanoma and presence of atypical melanocytes in the basal epithelium of the tissue sample [36].

There is no formal staging system for AM. However, the most commonly described system for AM in previous studies is the Ballantye clinical system which has three stages as follows: Stage I – localized disease, Stage II – presence of inguinal or pelvic lymph nodes and stage III – distant metastasis [37–39]. Interestingly, a recent study by Nagarajan et al. involving 160 AM patients found that the clinical American Joint Cancer Committee (AJCC) staging system (8th edition) for CM significantly stratified disease-specific survival of AM patients. Moreover, the authors recommended slight modifications in the AJCC 'T' category criteria of staging for better stratification [40]. Hence, either of the two staging systems can be used to prognosticate the disease in patients with AM.

7. Treatment

The main treatment options for AM are surgery, chemotherapy, radiation therapy and targeted therapies. According to a study which analyzed data of 1333 AM patients from National Cancer Database from 2004 to 2015, the authors found that surgery alone (48.7%) was the most common treatment given to the AM patients [6]. The use of chemotherapy and radiotherapy was similar throughout the study period but there has been a rapid increase in the use of targeted therapies for AM in the last few years. In **Figure 7**, we have provided an overview of the management of patients with AM.

7.1 Surgery

Surgery remains the mainstay of treatment. Most of the previous studies recommend surgical excision for Stage I and II AM. However, the benefit of lymph node

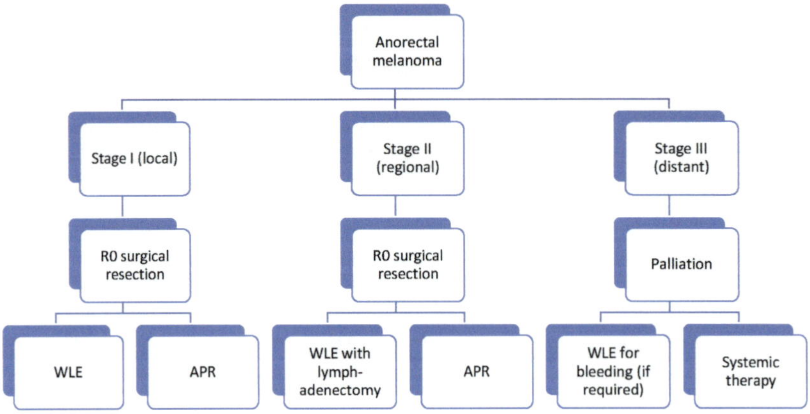

Figure 7.
A suggested algorithm for the management of anorectal melanoma. (WLE—Wide local excision, APR—Abdominoperineal resection, systemic therapy—Chemotherapy, targeted therapies).

dissection in AM has not been established. Unlike rectal adenocarcinoma and CM, lymph nodal metastasis has no significant impact on the long-term survival [41, 42]. The systemic dissemination of the disease occurs early in the course of the disease even before lymph nodal metastasis [43]. The 2020 UK National guidelines recommend R0 surgical resection in the least radical fashion [44]. Lymphadenectomy should be performed in cases with metastatic regional lymph nodes.

The main procedures for AM include: (1) function-preserving procedures such as endoscopic mucosal resection (EMR), wide local excision (WLE); (2) radical procedures such as low anterior resection (LR), abdominoperineal resection (APR). In a meta-analysis of 31 studies [43], 7 studies found APR to be superior to WLE [45–47], 11 studies found WLE to be better than APR [41, 48, 49] while 10 studies reported similar survival outcomes between the two procedures [42, 50, 51]. However, the local recurrence rate was significantly higher in WLE group (57% vs. 21.6%). The most recent study of 305 AM patients treated from 2004 to 2015 found no difference in overall survival (OS) between local and transabdominal resection (2.54 vs. 1.86 years, $p = 0.77$) [52]. Another recent meta-analysis found no significant difference in OS, disease-free survival (DFS) and local recurrence rates between WLE and APR on analyzing of data from 23, 7 and 19 studies, respectively [53]. So, we believe that WLE with regular surveillance should be the preferred approach. If WLE is not feasible or there is local recurrence without distant metastasis, then APR should be considered [39].

7.2 Chemotherapy

There is no standard chemotherapy regimen for AM due to the rarity of the disease. However, dacarbazine in combination with high-dose interferon and interleukin-2 was found to be effective in 10–20% cases of mucosal melanomas [54]. In a Turkish study of 6 AM patients, all patients received APR followed by adjuvant chemo- and radiotherapy [55]. The adjuvant chemotherapy included dacarbazine and temozolomide. In addition, two patients received ipilimumab, and one patient received interferon therapy. At the mean postoperative follow up of 12.5 months (6–26 months), 4 patients died due to extensive distant metastases while two patients were disease free [55]. In another study of 22 patients with metastatic AM, six patients received dacarbazine while one patient received temozolomide and thalidomide. The median survival in these patients was 9 months [56].

7.3 Radiation therapy

Radiation therapy has been used for palliation or in the adjuvant setting after organ preserving surgery such as wide local excision to reduce the chances of local recurrence. A study by Kelly et al. of 54 patients treated by WLE followed by hypofractionated radiotherapy reported good local control in 82% cases but the 5-year OS was only 30% [57].

7.4 Targeted therapies

Immune checkpoint inhibitors have become the standard of care in the treatment of metastatic CM. However, their role in MM is still under investigation. Cytotoxic T-lymphocyte-associated antigen (CTLA-4) and programmed-death (PD1) protein are the most common immune checkpoint targets expressed on activated T-cells with immunosuppressive effects. Ipilimumab is a fully human monoclonal that blocks the binding of CTLA4 with CD80 and CD86 ligands. It was the first agent approved for the treatment of advanced melanoma. It has an indirect effect on the T-cell mediated antitumor immune response. It prolongs survival in about 20% patients [58].

The ligands of PD1, PDL1 (B7H8) and PDL2 (B7DC) are expressed on tumor cells and other cell types. The immunosuppression of PD1 receptor is due to the interaction between T lymphocytes and tumor cells. PD1 blockage seems to be more effective toward t-cell activation than CTLA-4 inhibition. Nivolumab and pembrolizumab are humanized monoclonal antibodies against PD1. In a study of 44 MM patients having metastasis including 14 patients with AM, pembrolizumab was found to be more effective than ipilimumab in prolonging the PFS [59]. Another study reported the objective response rate of 23% and 37% in MM patients receiving nivolumab alone and in combination with ipilimumab respectively [60]. A study of eight patients treated by immunotherapy, one patient on PD-1 based combination therapy had stable disease and one patient with PD-1 monotherapy had complete response while rest of the six patients had progressive disease [35].

Mitogen-activated protein kinase (MAPK) pathway plays an important role in the cell survival, multiplication and differentiation. Overactivation of this pathway has been detected in various human cancers. Through this pathway many enzymatic kinases are expressed that are part of phosphorylation cascade including RAS, RAK, MEK and ERK kinases [61]. Overactivation of BRAF is one of the most common cause of abnormal MAPK signaling seen in cancers [62]. The MAPK pathway is activated in 40–50% cases of metastatic melanomas [63]. Hence, various BRAF and MEK inhibitors have been used for the treatment of metastatic melanoma.

Dabrafenib is a competitive reversible ATP inhibitor with selective BRAF inhibition. It has been found to be effective in 50–70% cases of melanomas with BRAF V600E or V600K mutations [64, 65]. Additionally, use of MEK inhibitors in combination with BRAF inhibitors such as vemurafenib plus cobimetinib or dabrafenib plus trametinib have prolonged PFS and OS of melanoma patients.

KIT kinase inhibitors such as sorafenib, imatinib, dasatinib, have been found to be very useful in the treatment of gastrointestinal stromal tumors. But they have not been very successful in the treatment of melanomas. However, some studies on KIT-mutated metastatic MM have shown good response to these KIT kinase inhibitors [66–69].

NRAS mutations are present in 15–20% cases of melanoma [70]. Tumors with NRAS mutations have aggressive tumor biology and show poor response to immune check point inhibitors [70]. MEK inhibitors especially binimetinib has shown promising results in phase II/III studies [71]. Several phase I/II trials testing the role of MEK inhibitors in combination with PI3K/AKT inhibitors are underway mainly including metastatic CM patients [70].

In summary, patients with AM, unlike CM, have poor response to targeted therapies. Also, the type of targeted therapy to be used depends upon the mutation analysis of the tumor as highlighted in **Figure 8**. However, the response rates with targeted therapies are better than conventional chemotherapy and are being increasingly used in clinical trials and oncology practice. Some immune checkpoints inhibitors and BRAF inhibitors are being used as adjuvant therapies in the ongoing clinical trials to reduce the recurrence rate after complete surgical excision.

7.5 Other therapies such as immune mediators such as interferon-a, interleukin-2

Studies have found alfa-interferon to improve relapse-free survival and overall survival in patients with CM. In CM, particularly in patients with positive nodal involvement, α-interferon at the dose of 20 MU/m2/day intravenously 5 day weekly

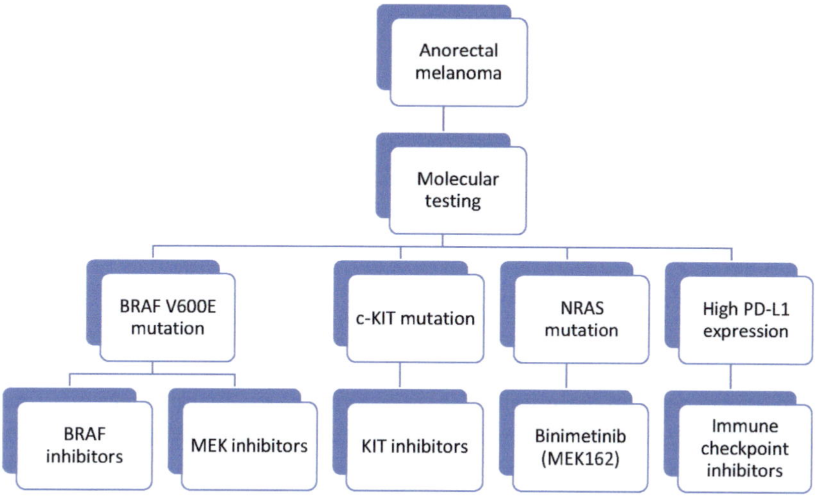

Figure 8.
A flow chart outlining the use of various targeted therapies for the patients with anorectal melanoma (molecular testing—Mutation testing can be done by immunohistochemistry or next-generation or high-throughput sequencing (NSG); BRAF inhibitors—Dabrafenib, vemurafenib, encorafenib; MEK inhibitors—Trametinib, cobimetinib, binimetinib (MEK162); KIT inhibitors—Imatinib, sunitinib, nilotinib; immune checkpoint inhibitors—Ipilimumab, nivolumab, pembrolizumab).

for 4 weeks, followed by 10 MU/m2/day subcutaneously three times weekly for 4–8 weeks had demonstrated a significant prolongation of DFS and OS [72]. However, their role in AM is not clear.

8. Prognostic factors

The 5-year survival rate of colorectal melanoma ranges from 4.3% to 17.4% [73]. The median survival of AM has been reported as 21 months [95% CI: 11–30] [15]. The 5-year OS rates of Stage I, II and III are 26.7%, 9.8% and 0% respectively [35].

A recent study by Menon et al. of 209 nonmetastatic AM patients found no significant difference in the median overall survival with chemotherapy (1.41 vs., 2.24 years, $p = 0.16$), radiotherapy (2.55 vs. 1.96 years, $p = 0.31$) and targeted therapy (2.07 vs. 1.96 years, $p = 0.95$) [52]. This study also found no benefit of adjuvant therapy in nonmetastatic AM cases after surgery. On the other hand, in 116 patients with metastatic disease, targeted therapy showed a trend toward higher survival (1.33 vs. 0.55 years, $p = 0.06$). On multivariate analysis, younger age, urban location of the patients and surgery were associated with better OS [52]. Other studies have found that age, tumor thickness, presence of ulceration, lymphovascular invasion, perineural invasion and tumor AJCC stage are the main predictors of survival [15, 39, 40].

The reported 1-,2-,3-,4-OS rates have been 67,40,40 and 32% in APR group and 100,100,67, and 67% in WLE group [39]. The median survival in WLE and APR groups were 36 and 13 months respectively [3]. In another study by Bello et al., no significant difference was found between WLE ($n = 81$) and APR ($n = 14$) provided the resection margins were tumor-free [74].

The site of origin of melanoma affects the prognosis as seen in cutaneous and mucosal melanoma. Whether the location of the tumor such as anal, rectal or anorectal affects the prognosis is not clear. In a study of 120 AM patients by Bello et al., the authors divided the patients in to three groups: anal (tumor below dentate line), anorectal (tumor at or traversing dentate line) and rectal (tumor above the dentate line). They found no significant difference in the DFS (23 vs. 28 vs. 27 months, $p = 0.887$) and

OS (22 vs. 28 vs. 27 months, $p = 0.696$) between the three groups [74]. Additionally, they found no survival benefit with adjuvant radiation or systemic therapy.

In the largest study of 60 Asian patients with AM, the authors found age > 70 years, tumor size more than 5 cm, tumor thickness more than 10.5 mm, lymph nodal metastasis, tumor invasion beyond deep muscular layer to be associated with poor disease-specific survival on univariate analysis. Among these parameters, only age > 70 years and depth of tumor invasion were independent predictors of low disease-specific survival [75].

9. Conclusion

AM is an uncommon malignancy of the anorectal region with high malignant potential. Early diagnosis and treatment are required to achieve good long-term results. Surgical excision remains the mainstay of curative treatment. AM shows poor response to radiotherapy and conventional chemotherapy. Targeted therapies, in the recent years, have shown promising results. Future studies with the use of a combination of chemotherapy, immune check point inhibitors, BRAF inhibitors, and MEK inhibitors are required to improve the long-term survival.

Conflict of interest

The authors have no conflict of interest to declare.

Author details

Rahul Gupta[1]*, Nalini Bansal[2], Houssem Ammar[3] and Jyoti Gupta[4]

1 Department of Gastrointestinal Surgery, Synergy Institute of Medical Sciences, Dehradun, India

2 Department of Histopathology, SRL Ltd., Fortis Escorts Hospital, Okhla, New Delhi, India

3 Department of Surgery, Sousse Hospital, Sousse, Tunisia

4 Department of Radiation Oncology, Swami Rama Himalayan University, Dehradun, India

*Address all correspondence to: rahul.g.85@gmail.com

References

[1] Cagir B, Whiteford MH, Topham A, Rakinic J, Fry RD. Changing epidemiology of anorectal melanoma. Diseases of the Colon and Rectum. 1999;**42**:1203-1208

[2] McLaughlin CC, Wu XC, Jemal A, Martin HJ, Roche LM, Chen VW. Incidence of noncutaneous melanomas in the US. Cancer. 2005;**103**:1000-1007

[3] Cheung MC, Perez EA, Molina MA, Jin X, Gutierrez JC, Franceschi D, et al. Defining the role of surgery for primary gastrointestinal tract melanoma. Journal of Gastrointestinal Surgery. 2008;**12**:731-738

[4] Hillenbrand A, Barth TFE, Henne-Bruns D, Formentini A. Anorectal amelanotic melanoma. Colorectal Disease. 2008;**10**:612-615

[5] Chen H, Cai Y, Liu Y, He J, Hu Y, Xiao Q, et al. Incidence, surgical treatment, and prognosis of anorectal melanoma from 1973 to 2011: A population-based SEER analysis. Medicine (Baltimore). 2016;**95**:e2770

[6] Taylor JP, Stem M, Yu D, Chen SY, Fang SH, Gearhart SL, et al. Treatment strategies and survival trends for anorectal melanoma: Is it time for a change? World Journal of Surgery. 2019;**43**:1809-1819

[7] Cote TR, Sobin LH. Primary melanoma of the esophagus and anorectum: Epidemiologic comparison with melanoma of the skin. Melanoma Research. 2009;**19**:58-60

[8] Jemal A, Siegel R, Ward E, Hao Y, Xu J, Murray T, et al. Cancer statistics, 2008. CA: a Cancer Journal for Clinicians. 2008;**58**:71-96

[9] Jensen C, Kin C. Black is the new black: Prolapsing primary anorectal melanoma. Digestive Diseases and Sciences. 2017;**62**:2991-2993

[10] Bharti K, Nguyen MT, Skuntz S, Bertuzzi S, Arnheiter H. The other pigment cell: Specification and development of the pigmented epithelium of the vertebrate eye. Pigment Cell Research. 2006;**19**:380-394

[11] Paolino G, Didona D, Macri G, Calvieri S, Mercuri SR. Anorectal melanoma. In: Scott JF, Gerstenblith MR, editors. Noncutaneous Melanoma. Brisbane (AU): Codon Publications; 2018. pp. 83-98. DOI: 10.15586/codon.noncutaneousmelanoma.2018

[12] Curtin JA, Fridlyand J, Kageshita T, Patel HN, Busam KJ, Kutzner H, et al. Distinct sets of genetic alterations in melanoma. The New England Journal of Medicine. 2005;**353**:2147-2153

[13] Curtin JA, Busam K, Pinkel D, Bastin BC. Somatic activation of KIT in distinct subtypes of melanoma. Journal of Clinical Oncology. 2006;**24**:4340-4346

[14] Tacastacas JD, Bray J, Cohen YK, Arbesman J, Kim J, Koon HB, et al. Update on primary mucosal melanoma. Journal of the American Academy of Dermatology. 2014;**71**:366-375

[15] Sarac E, Amaral T, Keim U, Leiter U, Forschner A, Eigentler TK, et al. Prognostic factors in 161 patients with mucosal melanoma: A study of German central malignant melanoma registry. Journal of the European Academy of Dermatology and Venereology. 2020;**34**:2021-2025. DOI: 10.1111/jdv.16306

[16] Newell F, Kong Y, Wilmott JS, Johansson PA, Ferguson PM, Cui C, et al. Whole-genome landscape of mucosal melanoma reveals diverse drivers and therapeutic targets. Nature Communications. 2019;**10**:3163

[17] Donizy P, Wu CL, Mull J, Fujimoto M, Chlopik A, Peng Y, et al.

Up-regulation of PARP1 expression significantly correlated with poor survival in mucosal melanomas. Cells. 2020;**9**:1135

[18] Dahlgren L, Schedvins K, Kanter-Lewensohn L, Dalianis T, Ragnarsson-Olding BK. Human papilloma virus (HPV) is rarely detected in malignant melanomas of sun sheltered mucosal membranes. Acta Oncologica. 2005;**44**:694-699

[19] Helmke BM, Deichmann M, Otto HF. Anorectal melanomas do not harbour the Kaposi sarcoma- associated human herpesvirus type 8 DNA. Journal of Medical Virology. 2001;**64**:47-50

[20] Malaguarnera G, Madeddu R, Catania VE, Bertino G, Morelli L, Perrotta RE, et al. Anorectal mucosal melanoma. Oncotarget. 2018;**9**:8785-8800

[21] Kruijff S, Bastiaannet E, Muller Kobold AC, van Ginkel RJ, Suurmeijer AJH, Hoekstra HJ. S-100B concentrations predict disease-free survival in stage III melanoma patients. Annals of Surgical Oncology. 2009;**16**:3455-3462

[22] Bosserhoff AK, Kaufmann M, Kaluza B, Bartke I, Zirngibl H, Hein R, et al. Melanoma-inhibiting activity, a novel serum marker for progression of malignant melanoma. Cancer Research. 1997;**57**:3149-3153

[23] Schmidt H, Johansen JS, Gehl J, Geertsen PF, Fode K, von der Maase H. Elevated serum level of YKL-40 is an independent prognostic factor for poor survival in patients with metastatic melanoma. Cancer. 2006;**106**:1130-1139

[24] Buzaid AC, Sandler AB, Cl H, Scinto J, Poo WJ, Clark MB, et al. Neuron-specific enolase as a tumor marker in metastatic melanoma. American Journal of Clinical Oncology. 1994;**17**:430-431

[25] Gupta R, Singh AK, Dhagam S. Metastatic anorectal melanoma. Journal of Gastrointestinal Surgery. 2020. DOI: 10.1007/s11605-020-04604-8 [Accessed: 20 April 2020]

[26] Winkler N, Rezvani M, Heilbrun M, Shaaban A. Utility of dual phase liver CT for metastatic melanoma staging and surveillance. European Journal of Radiology. 2013;**82**:2189-2193

[27] Matsuoka H, Nakamura A, Iwamoto K, Sugiyama M, Hachiya J, Atomi Y, et al. Anorectal malignant melanoma: Preoperative usefulness of magnetic resonance imaging. Journal of Gastroenterology. 2005;**40**:836-842

[28] Wang S, Sun S, Liu X, Ge N, Wang G, Guo J, et al. Endoscopic diagnosis of gastrointestinal melanoma. Scandinavian Journal of Gastroenterology. 2020;**55**:330-337

[29] Murali R, Doubrovsky A, Watson GF, McKenzie PR, Lee CS, McLeod DJ, et al. Diagnosis of metastatic melanoma by fine-needle biopsy: Analysis of 2204 cases. American Journal of Clinical Pathology. 2007;**127**:385-397

[30] Mikkelsen LH, Larsen AC, von Buchwald C, Drzewiecki KT, Prause JU, Heegaard S. Mucosal malignant melanoma—A clinical, oncological, pathological and genetic survey. APMIS. 2016;**124**:475-486

[31] Ben-Izhak O, Bar-Chana M, Sussman L, Dobiner V, Sandbank J, Cagnano M, et al. Ki67 antigen and PCNA proliferation markers predict survival in anorectal malignant melanoma. Histopathology. 2002;**41**: 519-525

[32] Chute DJ, Cousar JB, Mills SE. A norectal malignant melanoma: Morphologic and immunohistochemical features. American Journal of Clinical Pathology. 2006;**126**:93-100

[33] Helmke BM, Otto HF. Anorectal melanoma. A rare and highly malignant tumor entity of the anal canal [article in German]. Der Pathologe. 2004;**25**:171-177

[34] Kaunitz GJ, Cottrell TR, Lilo M, Muthappan V, Esandrio J, Berry S, et al. Melanoma subtypes demonstrate distinct PD-L1 expression profiles. Laboratory Investigation. 2017;**97**: 1063-1071

[35] Dodds TJ, Wilmott JS, Jackett LA, Lo SN, Long GV, Thompson JF, et al. Primary anorectal melanoma: Clinical, immunohistology and DNA analysis of 43 cases. Pathology. 2019;**51**:39-45

[36] Paolino G, Didona D, Clerico R, DE Vita G, Corsetti P, Ambrifi M, et al. Cancer surveillance series: Role of demographic aspects, altitude and latitude in the extracutaneous malignant melanoma in a residential study. Giornale Italiano di Dermatologia e Venereologia. 2016;**151**:133-139

[37] Ballantyne AJ. Malignant melanoma of the skin of the head and neck. An analysis of 405 cases. American Journal of Surgery. 1970;**120**:425-431

[38] Singer M, Mutch MG. Anal melanoma. Clinics in Colon and Rectal Surgery. 2006;**19**:78-87

[39] Nusrath S, Thammineedi SR, Patnaik SC, Raju KVVN, Pawar S, Goel V, et al. Anorectal malignant melanoma-defining the optimal surgical treatment and prognostic factors. Indian Journal of Surgical Oncology. 2018;**9**:519-523

[40] Nagarajan P, Piao J, Ning J, Noordenbos LE, Curry JL, Torres-Cabala CA, et al. Prognostic model for patient survival in primary anorectal mucosal melanoma: Stage at presentation determines relevance of histopathologic features. Modern Pathology. 2020;**33**:496-513

[41] Thibault C, Sagar P, Nivatvongs S, Ilstrup DM, Wolff BG. Anorectal melanoma—an incurable disease? Diseases of the Colon and Rectum. 1997;**40**:661-668

[42] Perez DR, Trakarnsanga A, Shia J, Nash GM, Temple LK, Paty PB, et al. Locoregional lymphadenectomy in the surgical management of anorectal melanoma. Annals of Surgical Oncology. 2013;**20**:2339-2344

[43] Matsuda A, Miyashita M, Matsumoto S, Takahashi G, Matsutani T, Yamada T, et al. Abdominoperineal resection provides better local control but equivalent overall survival to local excision of anorectal malignant melanoma: A systematic review. Annals of Surgery. 2015;**261**:670-677

[44] Smith HG, Bagwan I, Board RE, Capper S, Coupland SE, Glen J, et al. Ano-uro-genital mucosal melanoma UK national guidelines. European Journal of Cancer. 2020;**135**:22-30

[45] Wanebo HJ, Woodruff JM, Farr GH, Quan SH. Anorectal melanoma. Cancer. 1981;**47**:1891-1900

[46] Ishizone S, Koide N, Karasawa F, Akita N, Muranaka F, Uhara H, et al. Surgical treatment for anorectal malignant melanoma: Report of five cases and review of 79 Japanese cases. International Journal of Colorectal Disease. 2008;**23**:1257-1262

[47] Choi BM, Kim HR, Yun HR, Choi SH, Cho YB, Kim HC, et al. Treatment outcomes of anorectal melanoma. J Korean Soc Coloproctol. 2011;**27**:27-30

[48] Ross M, Pezzi C, Pezzi T, Meurer D, Hickey R, Balch C. Patterns of failure in anorectal melanoma. A guide to surgical therapy. Archives of Surgery. 1990;**125**:313-316

[49] Zhang S, Gao F, Wan D. Abdominoperineal resection or

local excision? A survival analysis of anorectal malignant melanoma with surgical management. Melanoma Research. 2010;**20**:338-341

[50] Che X, Zhao DB, Wu YK, et al. Anorectal malignant melanomas: Retrospective experience with surgical management. World Journal of Gastroenterology. 2011;**17**:534-539

[51] Nilsson PJ, Ragnarsson-Olding BK. Importance of clear resection margins in anorectal malignant melanoma. The British Journal of Surgery. 2010;**97**:98-103

[52] Menon H, Patel RR, Cushman TR, Amini A, Seyedin SN, Adams AC, et al. Management and outcomes of primary anorectal melanoma in the United States. Future Oncology. 2020;**16**:329-338

[53] Smith HG, Glen J, Turnbull N, Peach H, Board R, Payne M, et al. Less is more: A systematic review and meta-analysis of the outcomes of radical versus conservative primary resection in anorectal melanoma. European Journal of Cancer. 2020;**135**:113-120

[54] Wang X, Si L, Guo J. Treatment algorithm of metastatic mucosal melanoma. Chinese Clinical Oncology. 2014;**3**:38

[55] Atak I. Anorectal malignant melanoma: Retrospective analysis of six patients and review of the literature. Prague Medical Report. 2018;**119**:97-106

[56] Ranjith S, Muralee M, Sajeed A, Arun PM, Cherian K, Nair CK, et al. Anorectal melanoma: Experience from a tertiary cancer care Centre in South India. Annals of the Royal College of Surgeons of England. 2018;**100**:185-189

[57] Kelly P, Zagars GK, Cormier JN, Ross MI, Guadagnolo BA. Sphincter-sparing local excision and hypofractionated radiation therapy for anorectal melanoma: A 20-year experience. Cancer. 2011;**117**:4747-4755

[58] Wolchok JD, Neyns B, Linette G, Negrier S, Lutzky J, Thomas L, et al. Ipilimumab monotherapy in patients with pretreated advanced melanoma: A randomized, double-blind, multicentre, phase 2, dose-ranging study. The Lancet Oncology. 2010;**11**:155-164

[59] Moya-Plana A, Gomez RGH, Rossoni C, Dercle L, Ammari S, Girault I, et al. Evaluation of the efficacy of immunotherapy for non-resectable mucosal melanoma. Cnacer Immunol Immunother. 2019;**68**:1171-1178

[60] D'Angelo SP, Larkin J, Sosman JA, Lebbe C, Brady B, Neyns B, et al. Efficacy and safety of nivolumab alone or in combination with ipilimumab in patients with mucosal melanoma: A pooled analysis. Journal of Clinical Oncology. 2017;**35**:226-235

[61] Graves JD, Campbell JS, Krebs EG. Proein serine/threonine kinases of the MAPK cascade. Annals of the New York Academy of Sciences. 1995;**766**:320-343

[62] Davies H, Bignell GR, Cox C, Stephens P, Edkins S, Clegg S, et al. Mutations of the BRAF gene in human cancer. Nature. 2002;**417**:949-954

[63] Eggermont AMM, Spatz A, Robert C. Cutaneous melanoma. Lancet. 2014;**383**:816-827

[64] Long GV, Trefzer U, Davies MA, Kefford RF, Ascierto PA, Chapman PB, et al. Dabrafenib in patients with val600glu or val600lys BRAF-mutant melanoma metastatic to the brain (BREAK-MB): A multicentre, open-label, phase 2 trial. The Lancet Oncology. 2012;**13**:1087-1095

[65] Ascierto PA, Minor D, Ribas A, Lebbe C, O'Hagan A, Arya N, et al. Phase II trial (BREAK-2) of the BRAF inhibitor Dabrafenib (GSK2118436)

in patients with metastatic melanoma. Journal of Clinical Oncology. 2013;**31**:3205-3211

[66] Satzger I, Kuttler U, Volker B, Schenck F, Kapp A, Gutzmer R. Anal mucosal melanoma with KIT-activating mutation and response to imatinib therapy- case report and review of the literature. Dermatology. 2010;**220**:77-81

[67] Hodi FS, Corless CL, Giobbie-Hurder A, Fletcher JA, Zhu M, Marino-Enriquez A, et al. Imatinib for melanomas harboring mutationally activated or amplified KIT arising on mucosal, acral, and chronically sun-damaged skin. Journal of Clinical Oncology. 2013;**31**:3182-3190

[68] Carvajal RD, Antonescu CR, Wolchok JD, et al. KIT as a therapeutic target in metastatic melanoma. Journal of the American Medical Association. 2011;**305**:2327-2334

[69] Guo J, Si L, Kong Y, et al. Phase II, open-label, single-arm trial of imatinib mesylate in patients with metastatic melanoma harboring c-kit mutation or amplification. Journal of Clinical Oncology. 2011;**29**:2904-2909

[70] Johnson DB, Puzanov I. Treatment of NRAS-mutant melanoma. Current Treatment Options in Oncology. 2015;**16**:15

[71] Ascierto PA, Schadendorf D, Berking C, Agarwala SS, van Herpen CM, Queirolo P, et al. MEK162 for patients with advanced melanoma harbouring NRAS or Val600 BRAF mutations: A non-randomised, open-label phase 2 study. The Lancet Oncology. 2013;**14**:249-256

[72] Kirkwood JM, Strawderman MH, Ernstoff MS, Smith TJ, Borden EC, Blum RH. Interferon alfa-2b adjuvant therapy of high-risk resected cutaneous melanoma: The eastern cooperative oncology group trial EST 1684. Journal of Clinical Oncology. 1996;**14**:7-17

[73] Tokuhara K, Nakatani K, Tanimura H, Yoshioka K, Kiyohara T, Kon M. A first reported case of metastatic anorectal amelanotic melanoma with a marked response to anti-PD-1 antibody nivolumab: A case report. International Journal of Surgery Case Reports. 2017;**31**:188-192

[74] Bello DM, Smyth E, Perez D, Khan S, Temple LK, Ariyan CE, et al. Anal versus rectal melanoma: Does site of origin predict outcome? Diseases of the Colon and Rectum. 2013;**56**:150-157

[75] Ren M, Lu Y, Lv J, Shen X, Kong J, Dai B, et al. Prognostic factors in primary anorectal melanoma: A clinicopathological study of 60 cases in China. Human Pathology. 2018;**79**:77-85

Chapter 5

Mucosal Melanoma of the Head and Neck: From Diagnosis to Treatment

Ullyanov Bezerra Toscano de Mendonça,
Júlia Guimarães Soffientini, Victoria Ficher Barbosa
and Keren Cozer

Abstract

Mucosal melanomas of the head and neck are very rare malignancies that present with aggressive behavior and poor prognosis. Usually diagnosed at advanced stages, thus presenting macroscopically as aggressive nodular neoplasms arising from the mucosa; few cases are detected in situ. Tumor staging for mucosal melanoma remains a challenge. Several staging systems have been suggested, including tumor-nodal-metastases (TNM) staging systems, but none are frequently used. There is no clear consensus on the management of head and neck mucosal melanoma, which reflects the rare nature of the disease and complexity of the anatomic site. The late diagnosis, frequently presenting at an advanced stage, denotes the aggressive nature of the disease. Currently, early detection and surgical excision is considered the primary method of treatment. The multidisciplinary team approach can help reduce morbidity and mortality once optimize treatment, reduce costs and minimize adverse events, while maximizing the chances of recovery.

Keywords: mucosal, melanoma, head and neck

1. Introduction

Mucosal melanomas of the head and neck are very rare malignancies that present with aggressive behavior, including frequent local recurrence, and poor prognosis. First described by Weber in 1859 [1] and classified as its own distinct disease by Lucke et al. in 1869 [2], they represent a small fraction of all head and neck melanomas.

Unlike cutaneous melanomas, which incidence is believed to be rising over the years, the incidence of mucosal melanomas seems to remain stable [2]. Its annual incidence rate in Europe was estimated in 1.5 per million, with slight female predominance (1.2 vs. 1.0 per million) and in people aged over of 65 years [3], with median age at diagnosis ranging around 70 years old – developing at more advanced ages when compared to cutaneous melanomas. Significant variation between races is observed, with the Japanese more likely to be affected (8%) when compared to Caucasians [4], especially regarding oral cavity mucosal melanoma, suggesting association of this particular subtype with common hereditary or environmental factors,

 IntechOpen

still not identified [5]. Mucosal melanomas represent 0.8 to 3.7% of all melanomas, 0.03% of all neoplasms [6] and occur most commonly in the head and neck (55%) [7], mainly in the nasal cavity (lateral wall and septum) and paranasal sinuses (ethmoid and maxillary sinuses) [6], followed by the oral cavity – approximately 80% in the mucosa of the upper jaws (maxillary anterior gingiva), in the keratinizing mucosa of the palate and alveolar gingivae [8] -, pharynx, larynx, and upper esophagus [3, 9].

To date there are no clearly established risk factors for the mucosal melanoma development [5]. Cigarette smoking seems to be a risk factor for the oral tumor, while exposure to formaldehyde has been suggested as risk factor for the sinonasal malignancy. Association with viruses, such as human papilloma viruses, human herpes viruses or polymavirus is unlikely. Although sun radiation is a well-established risk factor for cutaneous melanoma, there is no evidence of its implication in mucosal melanoma pathogenesis, since its common locations preclude exposure to UV light [3].

Another particularity of mucosal melanomas, divergent from the cutaneous ones, is the more hostile behavior and frequent neoplastic dissemination, which results in greater death rate [10]. The mucosal melanoma aggressive clinical course results in very poor prognosis, especially among old male patients, likely due to little understanding of this rare malignancy and delayed detection, given the lack of specific clinical features for diagnosis, a challenging scenario for clinicians and pathologists [4]. Studies made on European cases diagnosed between 2000 and 2007 showed survival rates in 1, 3 and 5 years of 63%, 30% and 20%, respectively, as well as high rates of locoregional recurrence and distant metastasis [3, 11].

Tumor arising from the respiratory mucosa (such as the nasal cavity) have different clinical and pathological features when compared to those involving oral mucosa, as melanomas originating from non-squamous mucosa behave differently than those originating from multilayered squamous mucosa [11], but still they share similar adverse outcomes and prognosis and, therefore, will be discussed further in this chapter [1].

2. Pathology and biology

Melanomas are malignant tumors arising from pigment cells - melanocytes. Tumors can either develop from stem melanocytes with cytogenetic variations or mature melanocytes with secondary cytogenetic alterations due to external stimuli [6]. Precursors of melanocytes migrate from the neural crest to their final destination through embryonic mesenchyme, along specific pathways, most of them ending up in the epidermis and dermis of the skin, while some of them can be found in other locations, such as the mucosal membranes of the respiratory, gastrointestinal, and genitourinary tract [2, 3]. Melanin, the main product of melanocytes, may be missing in rare cases (2 to 8%), resulting in a non-pigmented lesion, referred as amelanotic malignant melanoma [9]. The presence and the function of melanocytes in the mucosa remain unclear. A few studies have supported the hypothesis of anti-oxidative, antimicrobial and immunological functions [3, 6]. In the sinonasal region, melanocytes take part in the metabolization of polycyclic aromatic hydrocarbons, suggesting association between inhaled environmental and immune factors and the development of mucosal melanoma in this particular site [5].

The etiology and pathogenesis of mucosal melanoma of the head and neck is still not fully understood. Whether it is due to preexisting mucosal nevi or racial pigmentation affecting its site, no risk factors have been unequivocally linked to those features. Despite the common association between cutaneous melanomas and sun exposure, mucosal melanomas are associated with embryology alterations (justifying the close proximity of commonly affected areas), inhaled and ingested carcinogens (e.g. smoking and formaldehyde exposure) and family history. Reports suggest that smoking patients have greater prevalence of pigmented oral lesions due to a hyper-production of melanocytes in the oral mucosa. Furthermore, 33% of oral cavity mucosal melanomas are preceded by pathological oral melanosis - increased number of normal or atypical melanocytes in the basal cell layer of the oral epithelium. Even though, conflicting data suggest oral melanosis should not be considered a pre-cancerous lesion [6]. Molecular studies of mucosal melanoma show several genetic changes in intracellular signaling cascades, which may constitute the distinct pathogenic mechanisms among these malignancies. Genomic hybridization studies have shown varied chromosomal aberrations - gains of 1q, 6p and 8q; gain of function mutations, such as K642E, L576P, D816H and V559A; amplifications of the 4q12 locus [11].

Special attention is addressed to the high incidence of activating mutations in the c-KIT (CD117) oncogene, present in 80% of all primary mucosal melanomas, whereas it seems not to have pathogenic importance in cutaneous melanomas [2, 5, 11]. KIT is a transmembrane tyrosine kinase receptor, expressed on melanocytes, but also on hematopoietic progenitor cells, mast cells, primordial germ cells, and interstitial cells of Cajal. Activating mutations and amplifications generate activation of growth and proliferation pathways, which seem to be important and common in acral and mucosal melanoma, both tumors unrelated to sun exposure [8]. Screening for KIT aberrations may have diagnostic value, given the evidence of a possible pathogenic role of this gene in mucosal melanomas, as well as a possible a therapeutic target in these patients [12]. Therapeutic c-KIT blockade could be useful in the treatment of patients with activating KIT mutation [6]. New drugs, such as imatinib, work on this pathway [8].

Along its signaling pathway, Microphthalmia-associated transcription factor (MITF) is referred to be involved in melanocyte development. The amplification of this gene is found in approximately 15-20% of primary mucosal melanomas. RAS-mitogen activated protein kinase related genes overexpression were found in up to 90% of primary mucosal melanomas [11]. Mutations in B-type Raf gene (proto-oncogene BRaf), present in up to 70% of cutaneous melanomas, have been detected in less than 10% of primary mucosal melanomas [2, 11]. Differently from the Human Papillomavirus (HPV) infection, which leads to p16/INK4a overexpression, loss of p16 expression, CDKN2A mutations, and loss of heterozygosity are observed in up to 50% of primary mucosal melanomas. GNAQ/11 mutations were observed in only 9.5% of the patients, who also presented shorter mean survival when compared to patients with wild type GNAQ/11. Programmed death-ligand 1 (PD-L1) expression seems to occur less frequently in patients with mucosal melanoma, which may lead to believe that mucosal melanomas are less immunogenic due to a lower mutational burden [2]. Primary sinonasal melanomas develop due to distinct genetic abnormalities, that lead to diffuse activation of the PI3K/Akt and RAS-MAPK pathways. These specific genetic pathway alterations, however, are not associated with different prognosis [6].

The key molecular events that trigger the malignancy development and progression is still unknown, which makes it difficult to work on new specific or multimodal treatment for this disease [12]. We can observe that mucosal melanoma is one unique subgroup in a vast emerging molecular classification system of melanoma. The complete understanding of these mechanisms may hopefully lead to a future of more optimized target therapy [11].

3. Diagnosis

Melanomas are malignant tumors arising from pigment cells—melanocytes. Melanocytes in mucosal membranes are distributed to the oral cavity, nasal cavity, paranasal sinuses, esophagus, larynx, vagina, cervix, rectum, and anus [13].

Mucosal melanoma of the head and neck (HNMM) region constitutes 55% of all mucosal melanomas, but <10% of all melanomas of the head and neck region. A majority of these tumors are found in the sinonasal regions (55%), while the rest are located in the oral cavity (25–40%) [13–16]. Mucosal melanomas generally present at a later stage, are more aggressive and carry a worse prognosis regardless of the stage at diagnosis [17–31].

Of all mucosal melanomas, paranasal sinus has the worst prognosis. The best prognosis locations are the nasal and oral cavity [15]. In contrast to cutaneous melanomas, mucosal melanomas more frequently are amelanotic and present in a multifocal fashion [17]. Early detection provides the best chance at survival but is often difficult due to anatomic location [17, 22, 27, 29]. Mucosal melanoma remains a challenge for several reasons: firstly, the clinical diagnosis often occurs relatively late, because it is not usually confirmed before the disease is symptomatic; secondly, traditional aspects of cutaneous melanoma clinical staging may not apply; and thirdly histological diagnosis can be difficult due to its rarity and variable appearance.

3.1 Clinical signs and symptoms

Presenting symptoms of mucosal melanomas differ in relation to the site of origin.

3.1.1 Primary mucosal melanomas of the nose and paranasal sinuses

Sinonasal primary mucosal melanomas (PMM) account for <1% of all melanomas and <5% of all sinonasal tract neoplasms [32].

In the sinonasal tract, early signs and symptoms are similar to those encountered in inflammatory benign conditions and therefore may be overlooked for some time [33].

The tumors can present with non-specific symptoms including nasal obstruction, facial pain, rhinorrhea and epistaxis [34]. In advanced stage primary tumors, symptoms such as diplopia, exophthalmos, ophthalmoplegia, headache, skin infiltration and ulceration, can occur [11].

At endoscopy, MM may present as a polypoid, with strict unilateral involvement in most cases. Lesions may have different degrees of pigmentation, with the possibility of diversely pigmented areas within the same mass. It can assume dark, brown, red, or pale white colors.

Compared with oral melanoma, completely amelanotic tumors are rare but when they do occur are associated with an even worse prognosis because of a more aggressive biology and greater difficulty in diagnosis [33]. Furthermore, multiple lesions (satellite lesions) can be frequently observed, even centimeters away from the main tumor, with spreading occurring along the mucosal/submucosal planes.

Among sinonasal cases, approximately 80% are located in the nasal cavity itself, most commonly the middle and inferior turbinates, lateral nasal wall and nasal septum, while 20% occur in the paranasal sinuses [13, 15, 16].

Concurrent nasal and paranasal lesions are infrequent.

The most frequently involved paranasal sinus is the maxillary sinus followed by the ethmoid, frontal and sphenoid sinuses respectively [11]. Primary lesions of the sphenoid and frontal sinus are exceedingly rare [11, 35].

Most of the patients with melanomas of the nasal cavity (75%) are diagnosed with clinically localized disease. That is the reason why patients with nasal melanoma have a more favorable prognosis when compared with melanoma arising from other head and neck sites. However, melanomas of the paranasal sinuses are usually advanced at presentation. PMMs of the ethmoid and maxillary sinuses have a worse prognosis than those arising from other sites. This is related to the higher T classification and late symptomatology. When occurs infiltration into the orbit, skull base, infratemporal fossa or facial soft tissue, the outcome is very poor [36–39]. At initial diagnosis, lymphatic metastases are present in 10% to 20% of patients with sinonasal PMMs, and <10% of patients have evidence of distant metastases [40]. 40% of cases will develop distant metastases in lungs, brain, bone, and liver, during the course of the disease [41]. Vascular and neural invasion is observed in approximately 40% of patients [42]. Early and repeated recurrences is frequently noticed in malignant melanomas of the nasal cavity and paranal sinuses.

3.1.2 Primary mucosal melanomas of the oral cavity

Primary mucosal melanomas of the oral cavity account for <1% of all melanomas, 0.5% of all oral malignancies, and 40% of all PMMs of the head and neck. The incidence of oral PMMs is higher in Asians, Africans, Hispanics, and Asian Indians [43–45].

Oral primary mucosal melanomas tend to present late as they are usually asymptomatic in the early stages and are often unnoticed by patients [11].

Compared to sinonasal disease, it may be diagnosed earlier due to the greater accessibility for inspection and oral examination.

Oral MM generally presents as a hyperpigmented lesion (**Figures 1** and **2**), with a wide range of colors varying from black, brown, gray to reddish or white. Interestingly, oral lesions may be amelanotic in up to 10–30% of cases; in these patients, diagnosis may be challenging. Amelanotic melanomas may simulate pyogenic granulomas [46, 47].

The tumors can be macular, nodular or plaque-like. Just like cutaneous melanomas, melanoma in the mouth may be asymmetric with irregular borders.

There can also be non-specific symptoms including bleeding, ulceration and pain, which is associated with the vertical growth of the lesion [48].

Macular lesions are flat, and up to one-third of patients have a long history of mucosal pigmentation (melanosis) [49, 50], which is considered the radial growth phase before invasion of underlying tissues (vertical growth phase). Nodular tumors, conversely, have an irregular surface and present as ulcerated, exophytic lesions.

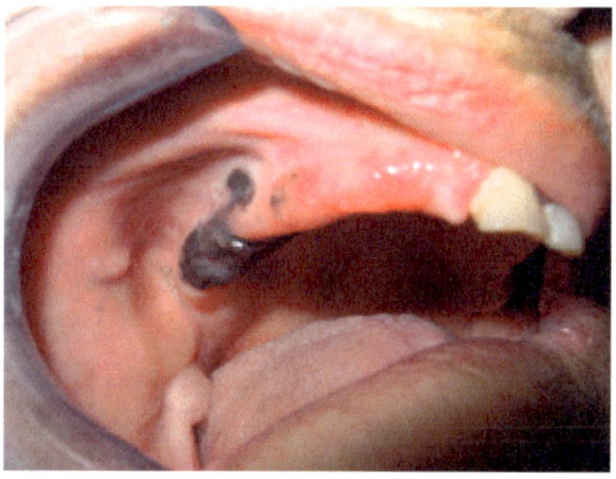

Figure 1.
Aveolar ridge mucosal melanoma.

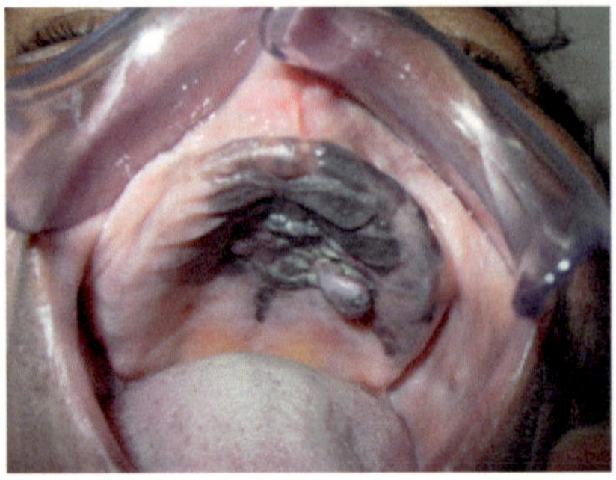

Figure 2.
Hard palate mucosal melanoma.

As with the sinonasal tract, it is also possible to observe satellite lesions in the oral cavity surrounding the primary lesion [49, 51].

The majority of oral melanomas occur in the maxillary alveolar ridge or the hard palate. Such locations favor early invasion of underlying bone, which may account for their poor prognosis. The buccal mucosa, lips, tongue, floor of the mouth, and uvula can also be affected as well [52].

The involvement of other subsites (floor of the mouth and tongue) is not commonly observed.

Tanaka et al. [52] featured oral MM into 5 types: pigmented, nodular type; non-pigmented, nodular type; pigmented, macular type; pigmented, mixed type; non-pigmented, mixed type. This classification was based in patterns of growth and presence of pigmentation.

25% of the patients with oral cavity melanomas present with lymph node metastases. The likelihood of cervical lymph node metastases increases when the tumor thickness is more than 5 mm [53, 54]. Wu et al. [52], on the other hand, found that MMs with a nodular pattern of growth have a higher risk of nodal involvement compared to macular melanomas.

3.1.3 Primary mucosal melanomas of other head and neck sites

Rare cases of laryngeal [55], oropharyngeal [56] and nasopharyngeal [50, 57] MM have been reported; these lesions are extremely rare, with only sixty cases reported in the literature. The tumors are most commonly located in the supraglottic region (62.2%) followed by the vocal cords (37.8%).

Clinical presentation does not generally differ from that typical of other primary tumors, mainly squamous cell carcinomas, arising in the same sites.

The symptoms of laryngeal MM are dysphagia, hoarseness, and painful sore throat [18, 19, 58].

Pharyngeal lesions may cause hemorrhage, dysphagia and/or dyspnea [19].

Symptoms of nasopharyngeal PMMs are similar to sinonasal PMMs; the tumors usually present with epistaxis, nasal obstruction, and obstruction of the Eustachian tube with serous otitis [19].

Notably, the risk of nodal (65.5%) and distant (59.3%) metastases in pharyngolaryngeal lesions is definitely higher than in other head and neck subsites [4].

As a general rule, the risk of nodal involvement in HNMM at presentation is higher in oral (25-43%) [47] than in sinonasal lesions (<10%) [35, 53].

The high rates of cervical node involvement at presentation is probably related to the size of primary lesions. 61% of nodal involvement occurs in lesions larger than 4 cm. Levels I (68%), II (68%) and III (23%) are the most commonly involved, whereas the frequency of metastases at levels IV (12%) and V (2%) is much lower [44]. The occurrence of distant metastases at presentation is low (5-10%), with no significant difference between oral and sinonasal lesions [53, 59]. The brain and lungs are the preferential sites of distant localization, whereas multiple organ involvement may be detected in up to one-third of cases [53].

3.2 Histological diagnosis

Head and neck PMMs are usually diagnosed at advanced stages, thus presenting macroscopically as aggressive nodular neoplasms arising from the mucosa; few cases are detected in situ [60]. Histopathological diagnosis is straightforward when the tumor cells are melanin rich. About two thirds of mucosal melanomas contain some intracytoplasmic brown pigment, which has to be confirmed as melanin and can be found in tumor cells or macrophages [61].

The histological features of HNMM can be as diverse as cutaneous melanomas [62], with variable mitotic activity and cell morphology [11]. Approximately 15 to 50% of cases presents with amelanotic lesions [63, 64]; as they can mimic another malignant neoplasms, including squamous cell carcinoma, this diagnosis has been challenging. These tumors frequently have a worse outcome [65, 66].

Histologically, mucosal melanoma is characterized by the proliferation of neoplastic melanocytes with variable phenotypes (epithelioid, spindle, and plasmacytoid cells without maturation and with nuclear changes, appearing as large and hyperchromatic nuclei with prominent nucleoli) that are arranged in a sheet-like, organoid, alveolar, solid, or desmoplastic architecture. They display high mitotic activity and show a pattern of invasion of the submucosa destroying the underlying tissues [67–69].

Tumors with mixed cell phenotypes are more related with vascular invasion and the development of metastasis. The neoplastic proliferation is commonly found along the junction between the epithelial and lamina propria, but this may be difficult to detect in advanced and ulcerated lesions [70].

Molecular studies have tried to find clinical predictors and immunohistochemical biomarkers to improve outcomes and survival rates.

Immunohistochemical stains may help distinguish mucosal melanoma from other malignancies and from cutaneous melanoma.

PMMs variously express S-100 protein and melanocytic markers, including MART-1/Melan-A, tyrosinase, HMB- 45, and MITF. 62 S-100 protein has greater sensitivity, but HMB-45 is probably more specific [42]. The absence or scarcity of melanin makes the diagnosis difficult and immunohistochemical techniques are required. The cells of amelanotic melanomas are positive for S-100 protein Melan-A, HMB-45, MITF and vimentin; and negative for cytokeratin [71].

One study assessed the expression of DNA mismatch repair and looked for the presence of microsatellite instability in HNMM. They showed that the cells had increased expression of mismatch repair proteins and increased microsatellite stability [72]. Besides these classical markers, the diagnostic potential of other molecules has been evaluated in Primary Oral Mucosal Melanoma (POMM), in particular several adhesion molecules. Integrin beta-3 and CD166 expression is correlated with extensive vascular invasion, while lower expression of CD54 is correlated with cell necrosis [73].

The expression of BCL2 in POMM has an important correlation with a longer overall survival [74].

The expression of podoplanin and CD13 in combination with S100 has been useful in the evaluation of lymph vessel and blood vessel invasion. Both markers are related to a poorer prognosis [75].

Programmed cell death ligand 1 (PDL-1) is known as a potent prognostic biomarker in several human tumors. Although this experimental evidence strongly supports the use of monoclonal antibodies targeting immune checkpoint proteins in MM, PDL-1 expression does not seem to be predictive of patient outcome, at least in melanoma [76]. Indeed, although PDL-1 positive tumors achieve a better responses to immunotherapies, PDL-1 negative patients can also have good outcomes.

3.3 Imaging of melanomas of the head and neck

When malignancy is suspected, computed tomography (CT) and magnetic resonance imaging (MRI) are valuable in defining the locoregional extent of the tumor, which is critical in determining resectability. For more accurate evaluation of MM, magnetic resonance imaging (MRI) is the modality of choice. This modality provide more information about the tumor, the localization, its relation to adjacent structures, and expansive or infiltrative characteristics. The analysis of signals in the different sequences is more.

sophisticated than the analysis of CT densities. The MRI signal of mucosal melanoma is influenced by the amount of melanotic pigment and hemorrhage within the lesion.

CT and MRI, when used together, can be complementary and define even better the invasion and destruction of structures of the skull base by soft-tissue masses.

The paramagnetic properties of melanin and of the free radicals produced by the metals ligated to the pigment itself account for a MRI pattern composed of T1 hyperintensity and T2 hypointensity [77].

MM usually manifests radiologically as an aggressive solid tumor with destructive characteristics related to compression or infiltration. The tumor causes bone destruction and invades adjacent soft tissues [13]. Thus, pre-treatment tumor mapping requires definition of tumor relationships with all surrounding anatomic sites and subsites. It is mandatory the accurate evaluation of involvement of intracranial structures and the surrounding vital structures such as cranial nerves or vessels, the anterior cranial fossa, the orbits, the pterygopalatine fossa and the infratemporal fossa.

Tumors arising along the Eustachian tube or in the nasopharynx can spread to the skull base at the foramen lacerum or along the tube to potentially reach the middle ear.

From a surgical point of view, key elements in the preoperative staging of mucosal melanoma of the oral cavity and oropharynx include depth of submucosal invasion, extension across the midline bone invasion and infiltration of deep space of the suprahyoid neck [77]. When the neoplasm reaches important anatomic crossroads, such as the posterior third of the hard palate, the pterygopalatine fossa, and the foramen ovale, perineural growth should be accurately evaluated.

MRI is the standard imaging modality for postoperative surveillance. Micrometastases may be radiologically occult. Because of the high fluorodeoxyglucose avidity of PMMs, FDG-positron emission tomography (PET)/CT may play an important role in the staging of PMM and in selecting the goals of therapy for patients with suspected metastasis or recurrence [78, 79].

3.4 Staging

Tumor staging for mucosal melanoma remains a challenge. Several staging systems have been suggested, including tumor-nodal-metastases (TNM) staging systems, but none are frequently used. TNM staging is only used for head and neck mucosal melanoma [11, 18].

The often concealed locations of mucosal melanoma result in frequent presentations of advanced disease.

In addition, unique to these anatomic locations are vast vascular and lymphatic networks in close proximity to the primary tumor, allowing for diffuse spread, with approximately one third of patients having nodal involvement at diagnosis [17, 21, 22, 24, 25, 29].

While different staging systems are in place for mucosal melanomas of different primary sites, Ballantyne described a three level staging system for classifying mucosal melanomas in 1970, which continues to be largely used:

Stage I: clinically localized disease;

Stage II: regional nodal involvement (cervical lymph node metastases).

Stage III: distant metastatic involvement.

Although its major advantage lies in its simplicity, this classification does not include depth of invasion or local tumor extension. The classification provides limited prognostic information as the majority of patients present with stage I disease [80].

To overcome these limitations, the pattern of tumor invasion has been studied in depth by Prasad et al., who reported that progression of the invasion at the microscopic level is associated with clinical worsening and suggests increased aggression.

They proposed microstaging as a prognostic marker, based on invasion of tissue compartments [81]:

Level I (in situ disease)

Level II (superficially invasive: melanoma invading up to the lamina propria)

Level III (deeply invasive: muscle, bone or cartilage).

The study evidenced a statistically significant difference in disease specific survival rates in levels I (75%), II (52%) and III (23%) respectively. However, this classification system is based on histological findings, the disadvantage is that it can only be used in evaluation of tissues following tumor excision, although invasion noted on pre-treatment imaging can be included.

The American Joint Committee on Cancer (AJCC) staging system for head and neck mucosal melanoma is often utilized, beginning at stage III. This focuses on the extent or size of the primary mucosal tumor using it as a predictor for outcome [82]. Mucosal melanomas are aggressive tumors, therefore T1 and T2 are omitted as are stages I and II.

TNM Clinical Classification:

T – Primary Tumor

TX: Primary tumor cannot be assessed

T0: No evidence of primary tumor

T3: Tumor limited to the epithelium and/or submucosa (mucosal disease)

T4a: Moderately advanced disease involving the deep soft tissue, bone, cartilage, or overlying skin T4b: Tumor invades any of the following: brain, dura, skull base, lower cranial nerves (IX, X, XI, XII), masticator space, carotid artery, prevertebral space, mediastinal structures

N – regional lymph nodes.

NX: regional lymph nodes cannot be assessed

N0: no regional lymph node metastasis

N1: regional lymph node metastasis

M – distant metastasis

M0: no distant metastasis

M1: distant metastasis

Stage Grouping

Stage III: T3 N0 M0

Stage IV A: T4a N0 M0

T3 ou T4a, N1, M0
Stage IV B: T4b, Any N, M0
Stage IV C: Any T, Any N, M1

A staging system should be valid as a prognostic tool to target treatment in terms of overall survival, but this system is not yet identified. At this point, tumor thickness greater than 5 mm, more than 10 mitotic figures per high power fields and/or ulceration has been suggested as independent prognostic factors [11]. To develop a uniform staging system a more thorough understanding of the prognostic factors is required [17]. This could facilitate comparisons of the results of different institutions, and help define the best therapy.

4. Treatment/management

There is no clear consensus on the management of head and neck mucosal melanoma, which reflects the rare nature of the disease and complexity of the anatomic site. The late diagnosis, frequently presenting at an advanced stage, denoting the aggressive nature of the disease. Currently, early detection and surgical excision is considered the primary method of treatment.

4.1 Surgery

Surgical treatment is the "gold standard" [80]. Wide excision with clear margins is the first goal in surgical management, once the complete surgical resection with negative margins significantly improves patient prognosis [83], whereas positive surgical margins have been associated with a higher rate of distant metastases, decreased survival measures, and a significantly higher risk of death compared to patients with negative surgical margins [84–86].

The incision depends on tumor site and size. Due to low rate of regional spread and the lack of effect on survival, elective neck dissection is not recommended. Neck dissection is mandatory only in cases of clinical or radiological positivity neck. Sentinel lymph node biopsy is not usually performed [80, 87, 88].

Surgical excision as a monotherapy should be reserved for patients with small tumors, localized disease and negative margins [89].

For sino-nasal mucosal melanomas, endoscopic techniques or external incision can be used [80, 90, 91]. In cases of oral mucosal tumors, a radical surgical resection with clear margins is the only curative option, and in cases of large masses, maxillectomy or marginal or segmental mandibulectomy is a possibility [11].

For laryngeal or pharyngeal melanomas, for complete resection is necessary total or partial laryngectomy or pharyngectomy [91]. The HNMM can be an aggressive disease and has high recurrences, demanding extensive resection surgery leading to disfigurement [80].

In most cases, complete resection is technically impossible without a destructive or disabling procedure, due to the proximity of the tumor to critical organs, but also because of the acceptable cosmetic result [36, 92], which frequently makes an adjuvant therapy necessary. Supplementary surgery can be executed for patients with recurrent disease and no evidence of distant disease [35, 90].

The National Comprehensive Cancer Network (NCCN, U.S.A.) guidelines emphasize that primary treatment should be surgical for stage III to IVA in the AJCC staging system but state that surgery is not recommended for stages IVB and IVC. These patients should be allocated in clinical trials or offered primary radiation therapy [93].

4.2 Radiotherapy

Radiotherapy (RT) is indicated to control local disease, positive surgical margins, or in case of palliative therapy. The addition of radiotherapy to surgery (adjuvant RT) may reduce the risk loco-regional recurrence without any impact on overall survival and disease-specific survival neither on the risk of distant metastasis [83, 87, 94–98].

According to the NCCN, adjuvant RT is indicated for patients with resected melanoma with high-risk nodal disease with four or more positive lymph nodes, lymph nodes of ≥3 cm and macroscopic extranodal soft tissue extension [93].

There is no clear indication of the appropriate evidence and the best radiation scheme.

Particle-beam therapy has also been used to facilitate the delivery of high doses to the residual tumor while minimizing exposure to the surrounding normal tissues, avoiding severe adverse effect in patients with tumors proximal to critical anatomical structures [99–101].

Primary RT alone has been advocated in patients with non-operable disease or a poor performance status [91].

4.3 Chemotherapy

The role of chemotherapy is minor compared to the biological and immunological systemic therapies [102]. The paucity of association of chemotherapy alone with improve overall survival led to its discontinuation as the election treatment for patients with metastatic mucosal melanoma. Therefore, chemotherapy is nowadays used as an adjuvant therapy in combination with other immunotherapeutic and biological drugs [103, 104].

4.4 Biological treatment

The selective inhibitors of various targeted (targeted therapy) have been approved since 2011 and include the BRAF inhibitors, dabrafenib and vemurafenib, the MEK inhibitors, trametinib and binimetinib and c-KIT inhibitors, which provides an attractive opportunity for developing adjuvant therapies for HNMM, mainly for patients with advanced locoregional or metastatic disease.

Vemurafenib, dabrafenib and trametinib are options for patients with BRAF V600 mutations who have unresectable or metastatic melanoma, mostly in combined therapy [3].

The selective inhibition of c-KIT alteration with, for example, the tyrosine kinase inhibitor, imatinib mesylate, has been revealed significant outcomes in patients with the K642E c-KIT gene mutation [27] whereas dasatinib, showed promising results in clinical trials in patients with L576P c-KIT gene mutation, once the KIT gene is mutated or present in increased numbers in mucosal melanoma [28]. Nilotinib is another selective inhibitor of c-KIT that does not require an active transport mechanism to enter cells [3]. Sadly, target therapy for c-KIT-mutated mucosal melanoma does not attempt the clinical reliability detected with BRAF-targeted treatment in cutaneous melanoma.

In clinical trials vemurafenib, a BRAF kinase inhibitor, has been showed greater efficacy and tolerability when compared to the chemotherapeutic dacarbazine [105, 106], as well as binimetinib, a MEK inhibitor (MEK162), administrated before or after immunotherapy with better overall response, progression-free survival, and disease control [107, 108].

4.5 Immunotherapy

A role for biologic treatment, as well as immunotherapy, has emerged over the last decade. Recent studies suggest that immunotherapy may confer survival benefit to patients with advanced disease.

Multiple prospective and retrospective studies support the use of the monoclonal antibody targeting cytotoxic T-lymphocyte-associated antigen-4 (CTLA4), ipilimumab, a promising immunotherapy [109], and the inhibitor of interactions of ligands PD-L1 and PD-L2 with its receptor, programmed death-1 receptor (PD-1), therefore blocking T-cell activation (anti-PD1 agents), nivolumab and pembrolizumab [110].

Nivolumab has been used as a promisor therapy in clinical trials. In patients with ipilimumab monotherapy-refractory or ipilimumab in combination with BRAF inhibitor-refractory metastatic melanoma, nivolumab showed a higher overall survival rate than standard chemotherapy [110, 111]. Furthermore, nivolumab in combination with ipilimumab has been shown a higher overall response rate then monotherapies [112].

Just like nivolumab, other checkpoint inhibitors, like pembrolizumab, have demonstrated more improvement in progression-free survival, toxicity, and overall survival than ipilimumab [113, 114].

Durvalumab and atezolizumab, other anti-PD-L1 antibody monotherapies, have not been very successful [115], whereas ipilimumab, nivolumab and pembrolizumab are standard options for unresectable or metastatic melanoma and may have potential as adjuvant therapy [3].

5. Prognosis

The prognosis of HNMM is relatively dismal, often due to late diagnosis, with 5-year overall survival rate of 25% [116–121] and higher rates of local recurrence and distant metastases than cutaneous melanomas [10, 122, 123].

Distant metastasis is the most common cause of treatment failure. The most common sites for distant metastases are the lungs, followed by the liver, bones and brain [124].

Local recurrence is frequent and commonly associated to positive surgical margins. Advanced age is associated with decreased survival [59, 83, 98, 124–126]. Present of distant metastases, advanced T-category, ulceration, vascular invasion, deep infiltration and male gender are associated with a poorer prognosis too [8, 97].

The multidisciplinary team approach can help reduce morbidity and mortality once optimize treatment, reduce costs and minimize adverse events, while maximizing the chances of recovery. A collaborative interprofessional team includes surgery, medical oncology, radiation oncology, radiology, nuclear medicine and pathology [127]. A multidisciplinary team workup will provide proper appraisal evidence based decision-making, and the most helpful treatment planning and care.

6. Conclusion

Mucosal melanoma is an exceedingly rare variant of cutaneous melanoma, with aggressive behavior and less favorable prognosis. This could be because of late diagnosis, patients' delay or the obscured anatomic site of origin. Unfortunately, because of its rarity, is poorly described and infrequently studied. Establishing guidelines for the clinical course of mucosal melanoma has been challenging.

The etiology and pathogenesis remain unclear. To date there are no clearly established risk factors for its development.

Primary tumor resection is the best treatment that also provides additional prognostic indicators. The type of surgical approach used is dependent upon the location and extension of the tumor, but the goal is negative margins with minimal cosmetic or functional derangements. Unfortunately, achieving melanoma-free margins is often compromised due to the anatomical complexity of the region and the close proximity of critical anatomic structures. Elective neck dissection is indicated for patients with lymph node metastases, especially in oral mucosal melanomas where there is an increased frequency. Adjuvant external beam radiotherapy is generally advocated with chemotherapy and targeted therapy being used for distant metastatic or unresectable disease.

Systemic treatment with immunotherapy can offer scope for modifying the course of the disease but response rates are lower and clinical research remains a priority. More studies and investigations are necessary to provide enough information and increase the survival rates.

Author details

Ullyanov Bezerra Toscano de Mendonça*, Júlia Guimarães Soffientini, Victoria Ficher Barbosa and Keren Cozer
Department of Otolaryngology-Head and Neck Surgery, Federal University of Rio de Janeiro-UFRJ, RJ, Brazil

*Address all correspondence to: ullyanov@yahoo.com.br

References

[1] Weber CO. Surgical experience and research, in addition to interesting observations from the Surgical Clinic and the Protestant Hospital Bonn. Berlin, Germany: G. Reimer; 1859. pp 304-305.

[2] Yde SS, Sjoegren P, Heje M, Stolle LB. Mucosal Melanoma: a Literature Review. Current Oncology Reports. 2018 Mar;20(3):28.

[3] Ascierto PA, Accorona R, Botti G, et al. Mucosal melanoma of the head and neck. *Crit Rev Oncol Hematol*. 2017;112:136-152.

[4] Green B, Elhamshary A, Gomez R, Rahimi S, Brennan PA. An update on the current management of head and neck mucosal melanoma. *J Oral Pathol Med*. 2017;46(7):475-479.

[5] Spencer KR, Mehnert JM. Mucosal Melanoma: Epidemiology, Biology and Treatment. *Cancer Treat Res*. 2016;167:295-320.

[6] Paolino G, Didona D, Macrì G, et al. Nasopharyngeal Melanoma. In: Scott JF, Gerstenblith MR, editors. Noncutaneous Melanoma [Internet]. Brisbane (AU): Codon Publications; 2018 Mar. Chapter 4.

[7] Chang AE, Karnell LH, Menck HR. The National Cancer Data Base report on cutaneous and noncutaneous melanoma: a summary of 84,836 cases from the past decade. The American College of Surgeons Commission on Cancer and the American Cancer Society. *Cancer*. 1998;83(8):1664-1678.

[8] Zito PM, Mazzoni T. Cancer, Oral Melanoma. [Updated 2020 Feb 21]. In: StatPearls [Internet]. Treasure Island (FL): StatPearls Publishing; 2020 Jan-.

[9] Paulo LF, Servato JP, Rosa RR, et al. Primary amelanotic mucosal melanoma of the oronasal region: report of two new cases and literature review. *Oral Maxillofac Surg*. 2015;19(4):333-339.

[10] Pittaka M, Kardamakis D, Spyropoulou D. Comparison of International Guidelines on Mucosal Melanoma of the Head and Neck: A Comprehensive Review of the Role of Radiation Therapy. In Vivo (Athens, Greece). 2016 May-Jun;30(3):165-170. Comparison of

[11] López F, Rodrigo JP, Cardesa A, et al. Update on primary head and neck mucosal melanoma. *Head Neck*. 2016;38(1):147-155.

[12] Toscano de Mendonça, U. B., Cernea, C. R., Matos, L. L., & Monteiro de Araujo Lima, R. R. (2018). Analysis of KIT gene mutations in patients with melanoma of the head and neck mucosa: a retrospective clinical report. *Oncotarget*, *9*(33), 22886-22894.

[13] Natarajan E. Black and Brown Oro-facial Mucocutaneous Neoplasms. Head Neck Pathol. 2019 Mar; 13(1):56-70

[14] PDQ Pediatric Treatment Editorial Board. PDQ Cancer Information Summaries [Internet]. National Cancer Institute (US); Bethesda (MD): May 21, 2020. Rare Cancers of Childhood Treatment (PDQ®): Health Professional Version.

[15] Panda S, Dash S, Besra K, Samantaray S, Pathy PC, Rout N. Clinicopathological study of malignant melanoma in a regional cancer center. Indian J Cancer. 2018 Jul-Sep;55(3):292-296.

[16] Lee JS, Lee H, Lee S, Kang JH, Lee SH, Kim SG, Cho ES, Kim NH, Yook JI, Kim SY. Loss of SLC25A11 causes suppression of NSCLC and melanoma tumor formation. EBioMedicine. 2019 Feb; 40:184-197.

[17] Patrick RJ, Fenske NA, Messina JL. Primary mucosal melanoma. J Am Acad Dermathology. 2007;56:828-34.

[18] Mihajlovic M, Vlajkovic S, Jovanovic P, Stefanovic V. Primary mucosal melanomas: a comprehensive review. Int J Clin Exp Pathol. 2012;5:739-53.

[19] Lourenço SV, Fernandes JD, Hsieh R, Coutinho-camillo CM, Bologna S, Sangueza M, et al. Head and neck mucosal melanoma: a review. Am J Dermatopathol. 2014;36:578-87.

[20] Bartell HL, Bedikian AY, Papadopoulos NE, Dett TK, Ballo MT, Myers JN, Hwu P, Kim KB (2008) Biochemotherapy in patients with advanced head and neck mucosal melanoma. Head Neck 30(12): 1592-1598.

[21] Carvajal RD, Spencer SA, Lydiatt W (2012) Mucosal melanoma: a clinically and biologically unique disease entity. J Natl Compr Cancer Netw JNCCN 10(3):345-356

[22] DeMatos P, Tyler DS, Seigler HF (1998) Malignant melanoma of the mucous membranes: a review of 119 cases. Ann Surg Oncol 5(8):733-742

[23] Hodi FS, Corless CL, Giobbie-Hurder A, Fletcher JA, Zhu M, Marino-Enriquez A, Friedlander P, Gonzalez R, Weber JS, Gajewski TF, O'Day SJ, Kim KB, Lawrence D, Flaherty KT, Luke JJ, Collichio FA, Ernstoff MS, Heinrich MC, Beadling C, Zukotynski KA, Yap JT, Van den Abbeele AD, Demetri GD, Fisher DE (2013) Imatinib for melanomas harboring mutationally activated or amplified KIT arising on mucosal, acral, and chronically sun-damaged skin. J Clin Oncol 31(26):3182-3190.

[24] Hussein MR (2008) Extracutaneous malignant melanomas. Cancer Invest 26(5):516 534.

[25] Keller DS, Thomay AA, Gaughan J, Olszanski A, Wu H, Berger AC, Farma JM (2013) Outcomes in patients with mucosal melanomas. J Surg Oncol 108(8):516-520.

[26] Kim HS, Kim EK, Jun HJ, OhSY, Park KW, Limdo H, Lee SI, Kim JH, Kim KM, Lee DH, Lee J (2010) Noncutaneous malignant melanoma: a prognostic model from a retrospective multicenter study. BMC Cancer 10:167.

[27] Pandey M, Mathew A, Abraham EK, Ahamed IM, Nair KM (1998) Primary malignant melanoma of the mucous membranes. European J Surg Oncol 24(4):303-307

[28] Postow MA, Hamid O, Carvajal RD (2012) Mucosal melanoma: pathogenesis, clinical behavior, and management. Curr Oncol Rep 14(5):441-448.

[29] Seetharamu N, Ott PA, Pavlick AC (2010) Mucosal melanomas: a case-based review of the literature. Oncologist 15(7):772-781.

[30] Woodman SE, Davies MA (2010) Targeting KIT in melanoma: a paradigm of molecular medicine and targeted therapeutics. Biochem Pharmacol 80(5):568-574.

[31] Wu E, Golitz LE (2000) Primary noncutaneous melanoma. Clinics Lab Med 20(4):731-744

[32] Mendenhall WM, Amdur RJ, Hinerman RW, Werning JW, Villaret DB, Mendenhall NP. Head and neck mucosal melanoma. Am J Clin Oncol 2005; 28:626-630.

[33] Adisa AO, Olawole WO, Sigbeku OF. Oral amelanotic melanoma. Ann Ib Postgrad Med. 2012 Jun; 10(1):6-8.; Venugopal M, Renuka I, Bala GS, Seshaiah N. Amelanotic melanoma of the tongue. J Oral Maxillofac Pathol. 2013 Jan;17(1):113-5;

[34] Gilain L, Houette A, Montalban A et al. Mucosal melanoma of the nasal cavity and paranasal sinuses. Eur Ann Otorhinolaryngol Head Neck Dis. 2014; 131: 365-369.

[35] Moreno MA, Hanna EY. Management of mucosal melanomas of the head and neck: did we make any progress? Curr Opin Otolaryngol Head Neck Surg 2010; 18(2): 101-6.

[36] Moreno MA, Roberts DB, Kupferman ME, et al. Mucosal melanoma of the nose and paranasal sinuses, a contemporary experience from the M. D. Anderson Cancer Center. Cancer 2010;116:2215-2223.

[37] Loree TR, Mullins AP, Spellman J, North JH Jr, Hicks WL Jr. Head and neck mucosal melanoma: a 32-year review. Ear Nose Throat J 1999;78: 372-375.

[38] Dıaz Molina JP, Rodrigo Tapia JP, Llorente Pendas JL, Suarez Nieto C. Sinonasal mucosal melanomas. Review of 17 cases. Acta Otorrinolaringol Esp 2008;59:489-493.

[39] Roth TN, Gengler C, Huber GF, Holzmann D. Outcome of sinonasal melanoma: clinical experience and review of the literature. Head Neck 2010;32: 1385-1392.

[40] Rinaldo A, Shaha AR, Patel SG, Ferlito A. Primary mucosal melanoma of the nasal cavity and paranasal sinuses. Acta Otolaryngol 2001;121:979– 982.

[41] Medhi P, Biswas M, Das D, Amed S. Cytodiagnosis of mucosal malignant melanoma of nasal cavity: a case report with review of literature. J Cytol 2012;29:208-210.

[42] Barrett AW, Raja AM. The immunohistochemical identification of human oral mucosal melanocytes. Arch Oral Biol 1997;42:77-81.

[43] Dauer EH, Lewis JE, Rohlinger AL, Weaver AL, Olsen KD. Sinonasal melanoma: a clinicopathologic review of 61 cases. Otolaryngol Head Neck Surg 2008;138:347-352.

[44] Femiano F, Lanza A, Buonaiuto C, Gombos F, Di Spirito F, Cirillo N. Oral malignant melanoma: a review of the literature. J Oral Pathol Med 2008; 37:383-388.

[45] Sortino–Rachou AM, Cancela Mde C, Voti L, Curado MP. Primary oral melanoma: population-based incidence. Oral Oncol 2009;45:254-258.

[46] Sun C, Chen YF, Jiang YE, Hu ZD, Yang AK, Song M. Treatment and prognosis of oral mucosal melanoma. Oral Oncol 2012; 48(7): 647-52.

[47] Tanaka N, Amagasa T, Iwaki H, Shioda S, Takeda M, Ohashi K et al. Oral malignant melanoma in Japan. Oral Surg Oral Med Oral Pathol 1994; 78(1): 81-90.

[48] Douglas CM, Malik T, Swindell R et al, Mucosal melanoma of the head and neck: radiotherapy or surgery? J Otolaryngol. 2010; 39: 385-392.

[49] Lyu J, Wu Y, Li C, Wang R, Song H, Ren G et al. Mutation scanning of BRAF, NRAS, KIT, and GNAQ/GNA11 in oral mucosal melanoma: a study of 57 cases. J Oral Pathol Med 2016; 45(4): 295-301.

[50] Warszawik-Hendzel O, Słowińska M, Olszewska M, Rudnicka L. Melanoma of the oral cavity: pathogenesis, dermoscopy, clinical features, staging and management. J Dermatol Case Rep 2014; 8(3): 60-6.

[51] Hicks MJ, Flaitz CM. Oral mucosal melanoma: epidemiology and pathobiology. Oral Oncol 2000; 36(2):152-69.

[52] Wu Y, Zhong Y, Li C et al. Neck dissection for oral mucosal melanoma:

Caution of nodular lesion. Oral Oncol. 2014; 50: 319-324.

[53] Patel SG, Prasad ML, Escrig M, et al. Primary mucosal malignant melanoma of the head and neck. Head Neck 2002;24:247-257.

[54] Umeda M, Shimada K. Primary malignant melanoma of the oral cavity--- its histological classification and treatment. Br J Oral Maxillofac Surg 1994;32:39-47.

[55] Terada T, Saeki N, Toh K, Uwa N, Sagawa K, Mouri T et al. Primary malignant melanoma of the larynx: a case report and literature review. Auris Nasus Larynx 2007; 34(1): 105-110.

[56] Wagner M, Morris CG, Werning JW, Mendenhall WM. Mucosal melanoma of the head and neck. Am J Clin Oncol 2008; 31(1): 43-8.

[57] Bekci T, Aslan K, Günbey HP, Incesu L. Primary malignant mucosal melanoma of the nasopharynx: an unusual cause of unilateral hearing loss. J Craniofac Surg 2014; 25(6): e567-9.

[58] Aggarwal S, Kaushal V, Singla S, Sen R. Primary glottic malignant melanoma of the larynx (PGMML): a very rare entity. BMJ Case Rep. 2015:1-4.

[59] Bachar G, Loh KS, O'Sullivan B, Goldstein D, Wood S, Brown D et al. Mucosal melanomas of the head and neck: experience of the Princess Margaret Hospital. Head Neck 2008; 30(10): 1325- 31.

[60] Bridger AG, Smee D, Baldwin MA, Kwok B, Bridger GP. Experience with mucosal melanoma of the nose and paranasal sinuses. ANZ J Surg 2005;75: 192-197.

[61] Wenig BM, Dulgerov P, Kapadia SB, Prasad ML, Fanburg Smith JC, Thompson LDR. Neuroectodermal tumors. In: Barnes L, Eveson JW, Reichart P, Sidranski D, editors. World Health Organization classification of tumours. Pathology and genetics of head and neck tumours. Lyon, France: IARC Press; 2005. pp 65-75.

[62] Kim HS, Kim EK, Jun HJ, Oh SY, Park KW, Limdo H,Lee SI, Kim JH, Kim KM, Lee DH, Lee J (2010) Noncutaneous malignant melanoma: a prognostic model from a retrospective multicenter study. BMC Cancer 10:167.

[63] Satzger I, Schaefer T, Kuettler U et al. Analysis of c-KIT expression and KIT gene mutation in human mucosal melanomas. Br J Cancer. 2008; 21: 726-736.

[64] Song H, Wu Y, Ren G et al. Prognostic factors of oral mucosal melanoma: histopathological analysis in a retrospective cohort of 82 cases. Histopathology. 2015; 67: 548-556.

[65] Shiga K, Ogawa T, Kobayashi T et al. Malignant melanoma of the head and neck: a multi-institutional retrospective analysis of cases in Northern Japan. Head Neck. 2012; 34: 1537-1541.

[66] Thariat J. Poissonnet G, Marcy PY et al. Effect of surgical modality and hypofractionated radiotherapy on local control and survival from sinonasal mucosal melanoma. Clin Oncol (R Coll Radiol). 2011; 23: 579-586.

[67] Gondak RO, da Silva-Jorge R, Jorge J, Lopes MA, Vargas PA. Oral pigmented lesions: clinicopathologic features and review of the literature. Med Oral Patol Oral Cir Bucal 2012;17:e919– 24.

[68] Marcus DM, Marcus RP, Prabhu RS, Owo- nikoko TK, Lawson DH, Switchenko J, et al. Rising incidence of mucosal melanoma of the

head and neck in the United States. J Skin Cancer 2012;2012:231693. http:// dx.doi.org/ 10.1155/2012/231693.

[69] Smoller BR. Histologic criteria for diagnosing primary cutaneous malignant melanoma. Mod Pathol 2006;19:S34-40.

[70] Coutinho-Camillo CM, Lourenço SV, Soares FA. Head and Neck: Primary oral mucosal melanoma. At las Genet Cytogenet Oncol Haematol 2015; in press. Available from: http:// atlasgeneticsoncology.org/Tumors/ OralMelanomaID6647.html

[71] Prasad ML, Jungbluth AA, Iversen K, Huvos AG, Busam KJ. Expression of melanocytic differentiation markers in malignant melanomas of the oral and sinonasal mucosa. Am J Surg Pathol 2001;25:782-787.

[72] Marani C, Alvino E, Caporali S et al. DNA mismatch repair protein expression and microsatellite instability in primary mucosal melanomas of the head and neck. Histopathology. 2007; 50: 780-788.

[73] Bologna SB, Nico MM, Hsieh R, Coutinho-Camillo CM, Buim ME, Fernandes JD et al. Adhesion molecules in primary oral mucosal melanoma: study of claudins, integrins and immunoglobulins in a series of 35 cases. Am J Dermatopathol 2013; 35(5): 541-54.

[74] Prasad ML, Patel SG, Shah JP, Hoshaw-Woodard S, Busam KJ. Prognostic significance of regulators of cell cycle and apoptosis, p16(INK4a), p53, and bcl-2 in primary mucosal melanomas of the head and neck. Head Neck Pathol 2012; 6(2): 184-90.

[75] Wermker K, Brauckmann T, Klein M, Haßfeld S, Schulze HJ, Hallermann C. Prognostic value of S100/CD31 and S100/podoplanin double immunostaining in mucosal malignant melanoma of the head and neck. Head Neck 2015; 37(9): 1368-74.

[76] Fusi A, Festino L, Botti G, Masucci G, Melero I, Lorigan P et al. PD-L1 expression as a potential predictive biomarker. Lancet Oncol 2015; 16(13): 1285-7.

[77] Kim SS, Han MH, Kim JE, Lee CH, Chung HW, Lee JS et al. Malignant melanoma of the sinonasal cavity: explanation of magnetic resonance signal intensities with histopathologic characteristics. Am J Otolaryngol 2000; 21(6): 366-78.

[78] Haerle SK, Soyka MB, Fischer DR, et al. The value of 18F-FDG-PET/ CT imaging for sinonasal malignant melanoma. Eur Arch Otorhinolaryngol 2012;269:127-133.

[79] Lamarre ED, Batra PS, Lorenz RR, et al. Role of positron emission tomography in management of sinonasal neoplasms – a single institution's experience. Am J Otolaryngol 2012;33:289-295.

[80] Ballantyne AJ. Malignant melanoma of the skin of the head and neck. An analysis of 405 cases. Am J Surg. 1970; 120: 425-431.

[81] Prasad ML, Patel SG, Huvos AG et al. Primary mucosal melanoma of the head and neck: a proposal for microstaging localized, stage I (lymph node negative) tumours. Cancer. 2004; 100: 1657-1664.

[82] Sobin LH, Gospodarowicz MK, Wittekind CH. International Union Against Cancer (UICC). TNM classification of malignant tumours. 7th edition. Oxford, UK: Wiley-Blackwell; 2009.

[83] Ganti A, Raman A, Shay A, et al. Treatment modalities in sinonasal mucosal melanoma: a national cancer database analysis. Laryngoscope. 2019.

[84] Tajudeen BA, Vorasubin N, Sanaiha Y, Palma-Diaz MF, Suh JD, Wang MB. Sinonasal mucosal melanoma: 20-year experience at a tertiary referral center. Int Forum Allergy Rhinol. 2014;4 (7):592-597.

[85] Lee SP, Shimizu KT, Tran LM, Juillard G, Calcaterra TC. Mucosal melanoma of the head and neck: the impact of local control on survival. Laryngoscope. 1994;104(2):121-126.

[86] Penel N, Mallet Y, Mirabel X, Van JT, Lefebvre J-L. Primary mucosal melanoma of head and neck: prognostic value of clear margins. Laryngoscope. 2006;116(6):993-995

[87] Benlyazid A, Thariat J, Temam S, Florescu C, Choussy O, Makeieff M, et al. Postoperative radiotherapy in head and neck mucosal melanoma: A GETTEC study. Arch Otolaryngol-Head Neck Surg. 2010 Dec;136(12):1219-25.

[88] Amit M, Tam S, Abdelmeguid AS, et al. Approaches to regional lymph node metastasis in patients with head and neck mucosal melanoma. Cancer. 2018;124(3):514-520.

[89] Amit M, Na'ara S, Hanna EY. Contemporary treatment approaches to sinonasal mucosal melanoma. Curr Oncol Rep. 2018;20(2):10.

[90] Castelnuovo P, Turri-Zanoni M, Battaglia P et al. Sinonasal malignancies of the anterior skull base: Histology-driven treatment strategies. *Otolaryngol Clin North Am.*2016; 49: 183-200.

[91] Lazarev S, Gupta V, Hu K, Harrison LB and Bakst R: Mucosal melanoma of the head and neck: a systematic review of the literature. Int J Radiation Oncol Biol Phys *90(5)*: 1108-1118, 2014.

[92] Dauer EH, Lewis JE, Rohlinger AL, Weaver AL and Olsen KD: Sinonasal melanoma: a clinicopathologic review of 61 cases. Otolaryngol Head Neck Surg *138*: 347-352, 2008.

[93] http://www.nccn.org/professionals/physician_gls/f_guidelines.asp#site

[94] Wushou A, Zhao YJ. The management and site-specific prognostic factors of primary oral mucosal malignant melanoma. J Craniofac Surg 2015;26: 430-434.

[95] Wushou A, Hou J, Zhao Y-J, Miao X-C. Postoperative adjuvant radiotherapy improves loco-regional recurrence of head and neck mucosal melanoma. J Craniomaxillofac Surg 2015;43:553-558.

[96] Li W, Yu Y, Wang H, Yan A, Jiang X. Evaluation of the prognostic impact of postoperative adjuvant radiotherapy on head and neck mucosal melanoma: a meta-analysis. BMC Cancer 2015;15:758

[97] Lawaetz M, Birch–Johansen F, Friis S, et al. Primary mucosal melanoma of the head and neck in Denmark, 1982-2012: demographic and clinical aspects. A retrospective DAHANCA study. Acta Oncol 2016;55:1001-1008.

[98] Samstein RM, Carvajal RD, Postow MA, et al. Localized sinonasal mucosal melanoma: outcomes and associations with stage, radiotherapy, and positron emission tomography response. Head Neck. 2016;38(9):1310-1317.

[99] Zenda S, Kawashima M, Nishio T, et al. Proton beam therapy as a nonsurgical approach to mucosal melanoma of the head and neck: a pilot study. Int J Radiat Oncol Biol Phys. 2011;81(1):135-139.

[100] Yanagi T, Mizoe J-E, Hasegawa A, et al. Mucosal malignant melanoma of the head and neck treated by carbon ion radiotherapy. Int J Radiat Oncol Biol Phys. 2009;74(1):15-20.

[101] Mizoe J-E, Hasegawa A, Jingu K, et al. Results of carbon ion radiotherapy for head and neck cancer. Radiother Oncol. 2012;103 (1):32-37.

[102] Chapman PB, Einhorn LH, Meyers ML, et al. Phase III multicenter randomized trial of the dartmouth regimen versus dacarbazine in patients with metastatic melanoma. J Clin Oncol. 1999;17(9):2745.

[103] Tyrrell H, Payne M. Combatting mucosal melanoma: recent advances and future perspectives. Melanoma Manag. 2018;5(3):MMT11.

[104] Amit M, Tam S, Abdelmeguid AS, et al. Role of adjuvant treatment in sinonasal mucosal melanoma. J Neurol Surg B Skull Base. 2017;78(6):512-518.

[105] Larkin J, Del Vecchio M, Ascierto PA, et al. Vemurafenib in patients with BRAFV600 mutated metastatic melanoma: an open-label, multicentre, safety study. Lancet Oncol. 2014;15(4):436-444.

[106] Chapman PB, Hauschild A, Robert C, et al. Improved survival with vemurafenib in melanoma with BRAF V600E mutation. N Engl J Med. 2011;364(26):2507-2516.

[107] Ascierto PA, Schadendorf D, Berking C, et al. MEK162 for patients with advanced melanoma harbouring NRAS or Val600 BRAF mutations: a non-randomised, open-label Phase 2 study. Lancet Oncol. 2013;14(3):249-256. doi:10.1016/S1470-2045(13)70024-X

[108] Flaherty K, Arenberger P, Ascierto PA, et al. NEMO: a Phase 3 trial of binimetinib (MEK162) versus dacarbazine in patients with untreated or progressed after first-line immunotherapy unresectable or metastatic NRAS -mutant cutaneous melanoma. J Clin Oncol. 2014;32(15_suppl): TPS9102–TPS9102.

[109] Schadendorf D, Hodi FS, Robert C, et al. Pooled analysis of long-term survival data from Phase II and Phase III trials of ipilimumab in unresectable or metastatic melanoma. J Clin Oncol. 2015;33 (17):1889-1894.

[110] Robert C, Long GV, Brady B, et al. Nivolumab in previously untreated melanoma without BRAF mutation. N Engl J Med. 2015;372(4):320-330.

[111] Weber JS, D'Angelo SP, Minor D, et al. Nivolumab versus chemotherapy in patients with advanced melanoma who progressed after anti-CTLA-4 treatment (CheckMate 037): a randomised, controlled, open-label, phase 3 trial. Lancet Oncol. 2015;16(4):375-384.

[112] D'Angelo SP, Larkin J, Sosman JA, et al. Efficacy and safety of nivolumab alone or in combination with ipilimumab in patients with mucosal melanoma: a pooled analysis. J Clin Oncol. 2017;35 (2):226-235.

[113] Robert C, Schachter J, Long GV, et al. Pembrolizumab versus ipilimumab in advanced melanoma. N Engl J Med. 2015;372 (26):2521-2532.

[114] Ribas A, Puzanov I, Dummer R, et al. Pembrolizumab versus investigator-choice chemotherapy for ipilimumab-refractory melanoma (KEYNOTE-002): a randomised, controlled, phase 2 trial. Lancet Oncol. 2015;16(8):908-918.

[115] Redman JM, Gibney GT, Atkins MB. Advances in immunotherapy for melanoma. BMC Med. 2016;14(1):20.

[116] Gal TJ, Silver N, Huang B. Demographics and treatment trends in sinonasal mucosal melanoma. Laryngoscope 2011;121:2026-2033.

[117] Kingdom TT, Kaplan MJ. Mucosal melanoma of the nasal cavity

and paranasal sinuses. Head Neck 1995;17:184-189.

[118] Nakashima JP, Vi_egas CM, Fassizoli AL, et al. Postoperative adjuvant radiation therapy in the treatment of primary head and neck mucosal melanomas. ORL J Otorhinolaryngol Relat Spec 2008;70:344-351.

[119] Owens JM, Roberts DB, Myers JN. The role of postoperative adjuvant radiation therapy in the treatment of mucosal melanomas of the head and neck region. Arch Otolaryngol Head Neck Surg 2003;129:864-868.

[120] Temam S, Mamelle G, Marandas P, et al. Postoperative radiotherapy for primary mucosal melanoma of the head and neck. Cancer 2005;103: 313-319.

[121] Yii NW, Eisen T, Nicolson M, et al. Mucosal malignant melanoma of the head and neck: the Marsden experience over half a century. Clin Oncol (R Coll Radiol) 2003;15:199-204.

[122] MoriM, Sugiura M, Kono M, Matsumoto T, Sawada M, Yokota K, Yasue S, Shibata S, Sakakibara A, Nakamura S, Tomita Y, Akiyama M (2013) Clinico-pathologic analysis of 66 Japanese thin melanomas with metastasis of sentinel or regional lymph node. J Cutan Pathol 20:1027-34

[123] Thompson LD, Wieneke JA, Miettinen M (2003) Sinonasal tract and nasopharyngeal melanomas: a clinicopathologic study of 115 cases with a proposed staging system. Am J Surg Pathol 27(5):594-611

[124] Amit M, Tam S, Abdelmeguid AS, et al. Patterns of treatment failure in patients with sinonasal mucosal melanoma. Ann Surg Oncol. 2018;25(6):1723-1729.

[125] Konuthula N, Khan MN, Parasher A, et al. The presentation and outcomes of mucosal melanoma in 695 patients. Int Forum Allergy Rhinol. 2017;7(1):99-105.

[126] Low CM, Price DL, Moore EJ, et al. Nodal and distant metastases in sinonasal mucosal melanoma: a population-based analysis. Laryngoscope. 2019.

[127] Mazzaferro V, Majno P. Principles for the best multidisciplinary meetings. Lancet Oncol. 2011;12(4):323-325.

Section 2

New Advances in the Mechanisms and Treatment of Melanoma

Chapter 6

The Role of the Meiotic Component in Reproduction of B-RAF-Mutated Melanoma: A Review and "Brainstorming" Session

Dace Pjanova, Ninel M. Vainshelbaum, Kristine Salmina and Jekaterina Erenpreisa

Abstract

The ectopic expression of cancer testis (CT) antigens and classic meiotic genes is characteristic and a hallmark of poor prognosis of melanoma disease. Here the potential mechanisms of meiotic influence on the cell and life cycle of malignant melanoma are reviewed in the genetic, epigenetic, and evolutionary aspects. The involved mutant B-RAF and N-RAS-induced senescence may be reversed by reprogramming, with stemness linked to meiotic landscape, possibly induced by DNA double-strand breaks at the mutual telomere hot spots. The induced by senescence mitotic slippage (reset of interphase from arrested metaphase) and resulting polyploidy trigger the meiotic ploidy cycle to function for effective DNA recombination repair, genome reduction, and escape of survivors, which enter the mitotic cycle again. The aberrant meiotic pathway in cancer is reviewed in the ancestral asexual variants; inverted meiosis is possible. The conundrum of cancer aneuploidy paradox, selection of fit clones, and the Muller's Ratchet of inevitable accumulation of harmful mutations is discussed. The bioinformatic study of the densely connected protein interaction network of CT antigen expressed genes revealed the melanomagenesis attractor composed of PRAME and small MAGEA group in primary tumors as compared with B-RAF-mutant nevi, restructured stemness network; invasive melanoma further displays the leading role of SPANX CT antigen group; meiotic genes are expressed in all three tissue cohorts.

Keywords: B-RAF-mutant melanoma, reversible senescence, reversible polyploidy, DSB hot spots, ancestral meiosis

1. Introduction

Approximately 50% of melanomas carry mutations in the gene encoding *B-RAF* [1]. Ninety percent of activating *B-RAF* mutations affect the codon 600 and the most common missense change there is V600E [2]. This mutation leads to a constitutive activation of B-RAF, and consequently of the MAPK/ERK pathway, promoting survival and proliferation of melanoma cells. Other frequent mutations in melanoma include *N-RAS* gene, which is estimated to be present in 13–25% of melanomas [1], and being upstream of the same MAPK/ERK signal transduction pathway. The MAPK/ERK signal transduction pathway involves a signaling cascade initiated by the binding of growth factors or cytokines to their respective receptors, resulting in activation of RAS, which then recruits RAF proteins, a family of protein kinases including B-RAF, to the cell membrane. Phosphorylation of RAF allows the activation of MEK1 [MAP kinase/extracellular signal-regulated kinase 1(ERK1)], which positively regulates the extracellular signal-regulated kinases (ERK). ERK can then directly phosphorylate downstream transcription factors, leading to increased transcription and eventual cell growth and proliferation [3]. Following the discovery of the V600E mutation, the pathway targeting inhibitor drugs was developed [4–10]. However, while initial responses are impressive, therapeutic resistance develops in nearly every patient at a median of 11–15 months of treatment [6, 7, 9, 11, 12].

Human nevi (benign lesions of melanocytes) also frequently harbor V600E mutation in *B-RAF* [13]; however, in spite of the oncogenic nature of this mutation [14], they display classical characteristics of senescence [15] and remain benign in the large majority of cases. At the same time, nevi are supposed to give rise to a quarter of all melanomas [16]. This led to the concept that oncogene induced senescence (OIS) precedes transformation [15, 17, 18], in particular if induced by mutant RAS or *B-RAF*. The expression of mutant RAS in normal human tissues inducing cell proliferation arrest was first described in [19] and further widely used as a model of OIS in normal cells. For a long time, OIS as well as senescence induced either by chemotherapy or oxidative stress (so called accelerated senescence ACS) were assumed as a barrier in premalignant tumor for tumor progression [20]. However, later it was found that senescence has also an opposite side and can reverse, so promoting cancer and metastases development [21–24]. Moreover, the cells that have experienced and evaded cellular senescence are more resistant to therapy than their counterparts [25]. The same group showed also that two different types of histone H3 lysine 9 (H3K9) demethylases, the flavin-dependent amine oxidase LSD1 and the 2-oxoglutarate-dependent Jumonji C family member JMJD2C, epigenetically disable oncogenic RAS- or B-RAF-induced senescence by enabling the expression of E2F target genes, which permits restarting of proliferation cycles. In turn, the inhibition of the H3K9 demethylases restores senescence and controls tumor growth of melanoma [26]. These experiments show the important contribution of the chromatin remodeling in OIS and cancer.

Biochemically, B-RAF has the same kinase activity as the serine-threonine protein kinase MOS [27] that is the main meiotic kinase [28]. Interestingly, proto-oncogenes c-ras and c-raf also participate in gametogenesis and when overexpressed (even non-mutant) can impose the meiotic mechanisms onto somatic cells [29]. In tumors, this pathway elaborating MOS-kinase can be triggered from mitosis through DNA damage checkpoint and senescence, supposedly providing them with the survival advantage [30–33]. At the same time, the expression of many germline proteins specific for meiotic prophase has been found upregulated in cancers [34–36] and in melanoma [37] as well.

Below we review the literature data of the abovementioned meiosis-associated processes and pathways involved in cancer (in the wide sense) and melanoma, in particular.

2. Senescence, TP53 function, and polyploidy in melanoma

Melanomas often derive from nevi, which already contain oncogenic B-RAF and N-RAS mutations. It was shown in several works that the melanoma genesis from these nevi is associated with the reverse of the OIS induced by these mutations. The mutual feature for all kinds of ACS (OIS, drug-, and oxidative stress-induced) is the introduction of DNA double-strand breaks (DSBs); a persistent DNA damage signaling was shown triggering senescence [38]. The response to the latter includes the activity of tumor suppressor transcription factor p53. Dysfunction of p53 is generally associated with malignant tumors and also with associated overcoming the polyploidy barrier [39]. In relation to melanoma, these issues will be briefly considered below. Wild-type (WT) p53 that is present at undetectable levels in normal tissues, when upregulated by DNA damage, is a potent inducer of apoptosis, cell cycle arrest, and cellular senescence, in general counteracting carcinogenesis [40], but also caring for stem cells by causing transient alternative splicing of POU5F1 in senescent embryonal carcinoma until the repair of DNA damage [41]. The tumor suppressor TP53 is mutated in its DNA binding domain in about half of somatic cancers [42]. In other cases, it is also mostly inactivated in other ways, e.g., by promoter methylation, etc. [43]. TP53 mutants, however, acquire additive functions, e.g., invasive features [44]. Melanoma is not an exclusion: with approximately only 10–19% disabling point mutations, WT p53 is found inactivated in approximately 90% of cases [45, 46]. The low frequency of p53 mutation in melanoma may be due to the overexpression of its counterpart oncoprotein MDM2, which is due to inactivation of *CDKN2A* locus encoding the dual tumor suppressors p16INK4A and p14ARF. Likewise, the most common somatic mutations associated with familial melanoma also disrupt the *CDKN2A* locus [47]. In the presence of oncogenic activation (B-RAF or N-RAS), p14ARF acts to directly inhibit MDM2, the major ubiquitin ligase that normally degrades and inactivates p53 [48]. The cooperation of B-RAF mutations with nonfunctional p53 in melanoma genesis was modeled by Patton and colleagues [49] in p53-deficient Zebrafish, where activated B-RAF induced formation of melanocyte lesions rapidly developed into invasive melanomas, resembling human melanomas and could be serially transplanted. Another tumor suppressor PTEN may also participate in melanoma genesis from B-RAF V600E nevi [50]. TP53 is a barrier to polyploidy [39], the latter is often reached by mitotic slippage (reset of interphase from arrested metaphase with a tetraploid genome). Mitotic slippage and thus polyploidization accompanies OIS or irradiation-drug-induced senescence in tumors with characteristic DNA damage response [51]; however, both senescence and polyploidy, induced by OIS or genotoxic treatments, can be reversed [52–55]. In this prolonged process occupying 7 and more days, the majority of giant cells succumb and the proportion of escape (de-polyploidized) cells may be rather low [56, 57] but they repopulate the tumor in the remote period of time. Mitotic slippage and DNA re-replication resulting in polyploidization was modeled in melanoma by Aurora A-kinase interference [58]. The DNA re-replication stress resulting in the fold-increased amount of DNA DSBs in the polyploidized cells was revealed. MDM2 antagonists relieved it by restoring the functional p53 and its downstream p21, interrupting re-replication of cells. Finally, the same was shown in melanoma: the experiments with prolonged expression of the oncogene N-RAS Q61K in pigment cells showed the induction of senescent multi-nucleated polyploid cells, however further overcoming OIS by the emergence of tumor-initiating mononucleated (de-polyploidized) stem-like cells from senescent cells. This progeny was dedifferentiated, highly proliferative, and anoikis-resistant, and induces fast-growing, metastatic tumors [59].

Besides inducing OIS, *N-RAS* and *B-RAF*-activating mutations can potentially impose meiotic features onto melanocytes (substituting by overexpressed B-RAF of meiotic MOS-MEK-kinase or alternatively triggering its pathway).

The possibility of imposing the meiotic (oocyte maturation) program by overexpressed RAS and RAF onto somatic cells was reported in literature [29, 60, 61]. Such trigger can supposedly favor the reduction division of polyploidized tumor cells [31–33] and likely also, in collaboration with REC8, the monopolar spindle of meiotic prophase [62]. In irradiated lymphoma cell lines, MOS was activated through polyploidy only in TP53-mutants, not their WT TP53 counterparts [30], where neither polyploidy nor MOS was induced. MOS protein was shown expressed in 20 types of cancer, including melanoma (https://www.proteinatlas.org/ENSG00000172680-MOS/pathology). As shown by more recent data on OIS in melanoma [58], the persistence of DNA damage in the absence of p53 function may be a bridge to invasive melanoma. And the persistent DNA DSBs in senescing polyploid cells, in turn, may be also a bridge from the G2M DNA damage checkpoint and/or mitotic slippage to the meiotic-type recombinative prophase possessing the same molecular background [33] (see also below in the section about SPO11 nuclease). So, B-RAF and N-RAS mutation, senescence with DDR signaling, deficiency of p53 function (upregulation of MDM2), induced and reversible polyploidy, and trigger to meiotic prophase are all molecularly related and this network can be potentially involved in melanoma genesis.

3. Cancer testis (CT) genes

CT genes were first defined as a group of tumor antigens that elicit a cytosolic T cell response and are expressed in male germ cells in the testis and various malignancies [63–65]. The first CT antigen identified was melanoma antigen 1 (MAGEA-1) [66]. Using the melanoma cell line MZ2-MEL and autologous cytotoxic T-lymphocyte (CTL) clones cytolytic to this line, MAGE-1 (subsequently re-named as MAGEA1, melanoma antigen A1) was identified as the target antigen for one of the CTL clones. This represented the first immunogenic tumor antigen shown to have elicited autologous cytotoxic T-lymphocyte responses in a cancer patient. Pursuing the same strategy, a range of other tumor-antigen genes, including MAGE-A3, another member of the MAGE-A family, as well as two additional families of antigens, namely the BAGE and GAGE gene families, were identified [64, 67–69]. The next huge step toward the identification of tumor antigens came from the screening of cDNA expression libraries with antibodies, the technology called SEREX (serological analysis of cDNA expression libraries) [70]. Very soon SEREX led to the identification of several categories of tumor antigens. To date, more than 80 families of CT genes are recognized and defined as germline restricted genes with evaluated expression in cancer [71]. As per today's definition, CT gene should simply exhibit a biased expression in the testis, ovaries [72], or the placenta [73], and in cancer.

CT genes can be divided between those that are encoded in the X chromosome (CT-X genes) and those that are distributed throughout the genome (non-X CT genes). CT-X genes are mostly members of gene families organized into complex direct and inverted repeats, and are expressed in testes primarily during the spermatogonial stage of spermatogenesis [74]. Annotation of the sequence of the human X chromosome has revealed that as many as 10% of all genes present on the chromosome are members of known CT families [75]. Further analysis of the expression patterns of genes of unknown function located in these repeated regions could even increase this estimate [76]. Melanoma has been found to have one of the highest CT antigens frequency expressions among other cancers. Moreover, higher frequency of CT antigens expression in melanoma is also correlated with worse disease outcome [77–80].

Our analyses of the NCBI's Gene Expression Omnibus [81] GSE98394 dataset including a cohort of 27 B-RAF-mutant nevi and 51 melanoma, described in details in [81] revealed the stark upregulation of many CT antigens in primary melanoma compared to nevi (Appendix Table 1). The densely connected component of protein-protein interactions (PPI) network of the upregulated melanoma CT antigens genes constructed using String Server [82] revealed the melanoma network module composed of 25 nodes, with a carcass of MAGEA-group hubs connected with the cohesin subunit SA-2 (STAG2) and the inhibitor of the differentiation-inducing retinoid acid receptor (PRAME) [83] hubs indicating to the acquired stemness (**Figure 1**). The high average node connectivity degree (5.84, PPI enrichment p-value <1.0e-16) characterizes this module as a CT antigen attractor of melanoma genesis from B-RAF-mutant nevi.

Similar upregulation of many CTA, however, different from those, occurs when the primary melanoma progresses and metastasis are formed as revealed in the TCGA-SKCM dataset that includes 103 primary melanoma and 368 melanoma metastases (https://www.cancer.gov/tcga) (Appendix Table 2).

The biological role of CT genes, particularly CT-X genes (a majority of them are CT antigens), in both germline tissues and tumors remains not well understood. However, studies have provided some evidence that MAGE gene expression may protect cells from programmed cell death and contribute to the development of malignancies by promoting survival [84]. It has also been shown that MAGE A2 is a strong inhibitor of the p53 tumor suppressor through histone deacetylase (HDAC)3 recruitment. In human primary melanoma cells, Mage A2 expression confers resistance to chemotherapeutic drugs by interfering with p53 acetylation [85]. Mage A2 interferes with p53 acetylation at promyelocytic leukemia (PML)-nuclear bodies (NBs) and with PMLIV-dependent activation of p53 through an HDAC-dependent mechanism, so downregulating it [86]. Usually, p53 is recruited to PML-NBs where it becomes acetylated and activated, and participates in the triggering of cellular senescence [87], a critical barrier against cell transformation (discussed above).

The mechanisms involved in the regulation of CT antigens expression appears to be promoted by DNA demethylation. Methylation of CpG islands within gene promoters is responsible for gene silencing due to both its effect on chromatin structure

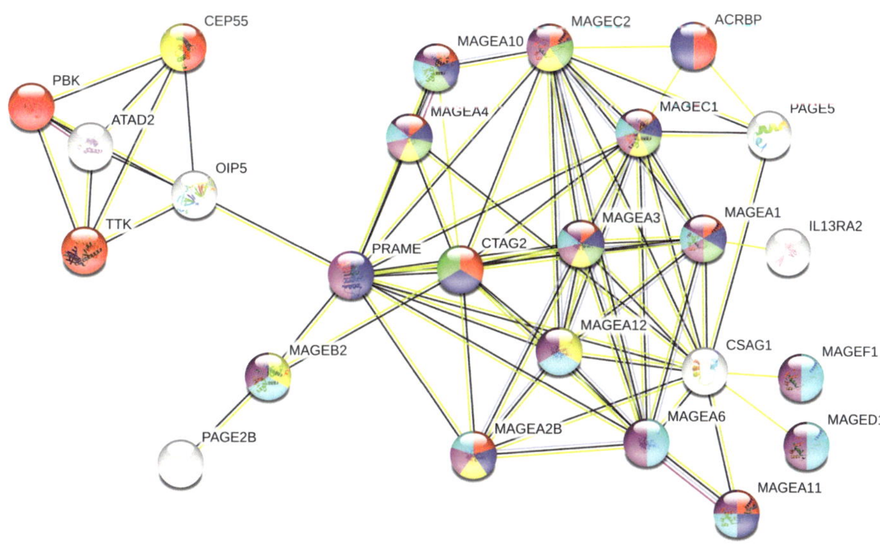

Figure 1.
The densely connected component of protein-protein interactions (PPI) network of the upregulated melanoma CT antigens constructed using String server [82].

and binding of transcription factors [88]. "Epigenetic reprogramming," consisting of concerted DNA pan-demethylation and corresponding chromatin remodeling, occurs twice in the human life cycle: during early embryogenesis and gametogenesis of primordial germ cells (PGC) [89]. So far, all CT antigens studied have methylated CpG islands in normal somatic tissues and are activated by demethylation during spermatogenesis [90]. Experimental demethylation of CT antigens promoters induces antigen expression in cells that do not normally produce them [91]. It has been proposed that the activation of CT antigens in cancer is a consequence of the ectopic induction of gametogenic program [74, 92, 93], which thus includes the meiotic component.

As recently found, all MAGEs contain a conservative E-ring domain and assemble with E3 RING ubiquitin ligases to form MAGE-RING ligases (MRLs) that act as regulators of ubiquitination by modulating E-ring-ligase activity [94]. The latter are acting at the cross-roads between tumor suppression and oncogenesis [95]. In addition, a majority of the CT antigens [96, 97] are intrinsically disordered proteins (IDPs). IDPs lack rigid 3D structures either along their entire length or in localized regions. Despite the lack of structure, most IDPs can transit from disorder to order upon binding to various biological targets [98]. Protein intrinsic disorder can serve as the structural basis for hub protein promiscuity; thus, CT antigens proteins can provide flexible linkers between functional domains [99]. Many normal cellular processes are associated with the presence of the right amount of precisely activated IDPs at right places and at the right time, those may be altered in disease, including cancer [100, 101]. The IDPs—features of the X-linked CT antigen-encoded genes, which can change their targets, as well as the relation of the MAGE group to ubiquitin-ligases suggest their highly adaptive post-translation functions for the cancer genome and proteome networks. This property is consistent with their activation by CTCF inhibitor and pan-genome activator, the CT gene Brother of Regulator of Imprinted Sites (BORIS) located at the chromosome region 20q13.2. This region is commonly amplified in human cancers [102, 103]. BORIS expression is normally restricted to testis and becomes aberrantly expressed in different types of cancer [104]. In melanoma, BORIS expression was observed in 59% of melanoma cell lines, in 16% of primary melanomas and in 34% of melanoma metastases [105].

Normally, BORIS plays a major role in regulating de-repressing, de-methylation processes during spermatogenesis—it removes imprinting from genes during the last mitotic division of type B spermatogonia producing the first spermatocyte [106]. In particular, in melanoma, BORIS binds near the promoter of transforming growth factor-beta 1 (TFGB1), a well-recognized factor involved in the transition toward an invasive state, activating it through transcriptional reprogramming [107]. BORIS is a paralog and antagonist of CTCF. A primary role for CTCF in the global organization of chromatin architecture was shown, which suggests that CTCF may be a heritable topological repressive component of an epigenetic system regulating the interplay between DNA methylation, higher-order chromatin structure, and lineage-specific gene expression [108, 109]. Nowadays, multiple studies have indicated an oncogenic role for BORIS [110–112]. Notably, emerging evidence has shown that BORIS functions as an epigenetic modifier in modulating the whole genome gene expression [113–115], including expression of other CT genes [116, 117]. BORIS was also found to be expressed in embryonal carcinoma, ovarian cancer [118] as well as cancer stem cell (CSC)-enriched populations isolated from epithelial cancer cells [119, 120]. The mRNA isoforms of BORIS genes are expressed in normal ovary and in the altered pattern, in epithelial ovarian cancer [121]. An association of BORIS expression with CSC-like properties was also observed [119, 120]. Moreover, it has been shown that BORIS association with the CSC-like traits occurs through the epigenetic regulation of *POU5F1/OCT4* [112]. OCT4 is considered a master regulator in the maintenance of stem cell pluripotency. Many studies have demonstrated a correlation between OCT4 and CSCs in many cancers, including melanoma [122–124].

In relation to metastatic melanoma, using the TCGA database (https://www.cancer.gov/tcga), we assessed the expression of a number of genes selected from the POU, SOX, SALL, and NANOG gene families with relation to stemness in normal and cancer stem cells [125] and noted an increase in stemness during transition from primary melanoma to metastases. Moreover, the heat map shows the reconstruction of the landscape in the expression of stemness-associated genes indicating to the whole genome rearrangement (**Figure 2**).

Melanocytes originate from the neural crest developing in embryo very early (as the fourth germ layer) and is associated with intensive cell migration. Melanomas in patients or cell constructs upregulating the Wnt pathway, associated with neural crest development, display epithelial-to-mesenchyme-transition (EMT) phenotype, worse prognoses in patients, and resistance to drugs in vitro [129]. The role of the neural crest development factors in ectopic regulation of melanoma was also investigated in [130]. Likely, because of the origin, nearly the root of the ontogenetic tree, melanoma is so invasive and malignant.

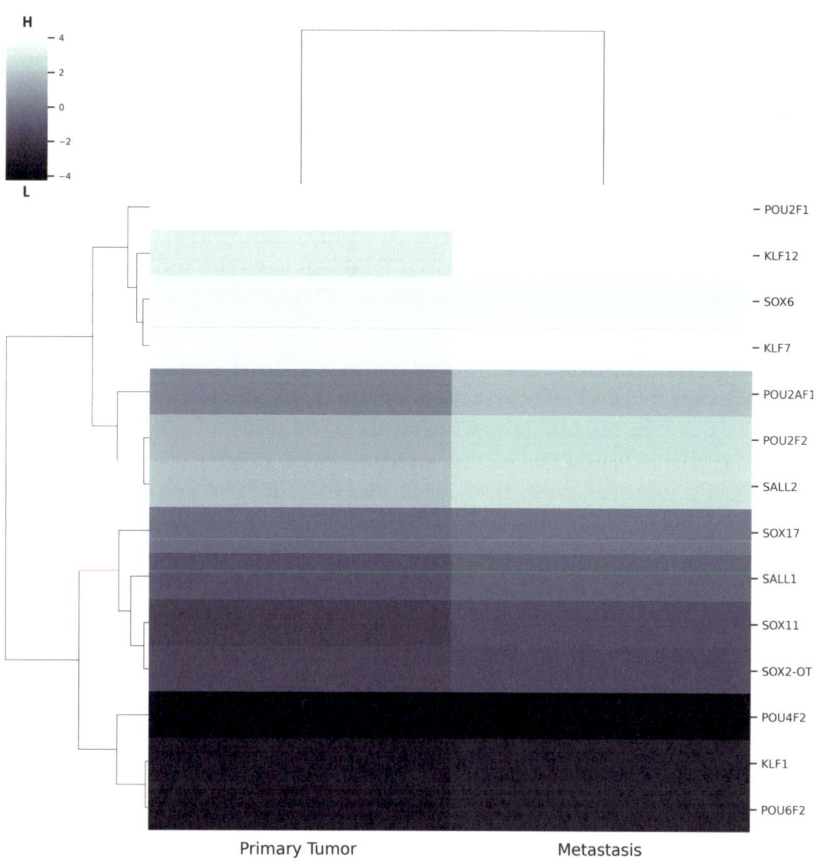

Figure 2.
Gene expression (in log2CPM values) of stemness genes in the cohort of 368 melanoma metastases compared to 103 primary melanoma from the TCGA-SKCM dataset (https://www.cancer.gov/tcga). The data was extracted from the TCGA database using the TCGA Biolinks Bioconductor package [126]. EdgeR [127] was used to perform differential expression analysis through the generalized linear model approach. The differentially expressed genes (DEGs) which were upregulated in metastatic melanoma (log2FC > 0, p < 0.01) were filtered for genes from the POU, SOX, SALL, and NANOG gene families with relation to stemness. Seaborn [128] was used to construct the heat map.

The particular interest for carcinogenesis represents the non-X CT genes or germline restricted genes that normally mediate meiotic program [30, 34–37, 131] and therefore are denoted by some authors, the meiosis-specific CT (meiCT) genes [36].

4. Conventional meiosis: in brief

The conventional meiotic progression is well described [28] and has been recently updated by Feichtinger and McFarlane [35]. Thus, only a short recitation of some of the main points is provided here.

Meiosis is a special mode of cell division that naturally occurs in mammalian only in the germ cells—in the male testis and female ovary. During meiosis, diploid germ cells undergo a single round of premeiotic DNA replication (4n), followed by two chromosome segregation events, meiosis I (reductional) and meiosis II (equational), creating haploid (1n) gametes. Meiosis I is marked by a prolonged prophase that is subdivided into five stages: leptotene, zygotene, pachytene, diplotene, and diakinesis, where during the first three stages, there occurs the formation of DSBs, homologous chromosome pairing, and synapsis and reciprocal homologous recombination (HR) between them. The initiation of meiosis is not fully understood in mammals, but it is thought that meiotic entry is initiated by upregulation of the stimulated by retinoic acid 8 (STRA8) gene expression—transcription activator that binds directly to the promoter regions of meiosis-specific genes [124–126].

During premeiotic DNA replication, a ring of specific cohesins is formed that holds newly formed sister chromatids together [127]. In meiosis I prophase, HR program is initiated by the generation of DNA DSBs along the chromosome axis in specific hotspots [128]. This is initiated by a protein complex, which consists of SPO11 and TOPOVIBL [129]. Generated DSBs serve as the substrates for the recombinase RAD51 and its meiosis-specific paralogue DMC1 acting as a heterodimer [130]. The hot spot selection in mammals mediates the zinc finger histone methyltransferase, PR domain containing 9 (PRDM9), which primes the DNA for DSB and exchange of DNA between chromosomes [131, 132]. Of note, in the case of meiosis, DNA DSBs are obligatory rather than the result of accidental damage, as in the mitotic cell cycle, and the recombination partners are homologous chromosomes in meiosis, whereas they are sister chromatids in DNA repair during mitosis. As the homologous chromosome bivalents after HR align on the metaphase I plate, the centromeres of sister chromatids form monopolar spindle associations. Loss of sister cohesion in the arm regions of chromosomes, but not the centromeric regions, occurs on entry into meiotic anaphase I permitting reductional segregation of homologous chromosomes. During meiosis II, centromeric cohesion is broken down and an equational segregation of the chromatids, like in mitosis, occurs [127].

5. Melanoma and meiosis specific CT (meiCT) genes

HR sites resulting in crossovers are initiated by the creation of DSBs in the leptotene prophase stage catalyzed by the protein Spo11 [132]. Spo11 is an homolog of the A subunit of type II DNA topoisomerase that together with TOPOVIBL, an homolog of B subunit, forms protein complex. The MREII exonuclease creates DNA nicks guiding the SPO11-TOPOVIBL complex to accurately catalyze DSBs along the genome in specific hotspots [133, 134]. Aberrant expression of SPO11 has been found in cell lines of melanoma and also lung cancer [135], see **Figure 3**, acute myeloid leukemia (AML) [136], cutaneous T-cell lymphoma (CTCL) [137] as well as in patient samples of melanoma, [135, 138], cervical cancer [135], gastric cancer [138], and CTCL [139]. Although the exact mechanism of SPO11 reactivation in cancer cells remains elusive, it has been shown that in CTCL, it is regulated epigenetically and temporary expressed at the onset of the cell division in G1/S phase transition [139]. This expression before DNA replication seems unrelevant but, indeed, it appears that SPO11 expression in B-RAF- and TP-53 mutant melanoma may be not dependent on the cell cycle phase (**Figure 3**).

SPO11 expression in CTCL cell lines decreased after cell line treatment with histone deacetylase (HDAC) inhibitors, e.g., Vorinostat and Romidepsin [137]. Moreover, SPO11-introduced DNA DSBs have also been shown to increase the risk of genome rearrangements and mutations in the germline [140]—a potential source of the idiopathic male infertility, which is associated with the 20-fold increased risk of the germline cancer [141]. Spo11 appears to be present in all sequenced eukaryotic genomes, and indeed it may be the only truly universal meiotic protein. At the same time, in many organisms, the recombination defect in Spo11 mutants can rescue meiosis by production of DSBs from an exogenous source such as ionizing radiation [142, 143]. On the other side, SPO11 was also found in species and tissues undergoing asexual life-cycles [143] or DNA recombination for nonsexual function. e.g., SPO11 was revealed in mouse germinal center B cells undergoing

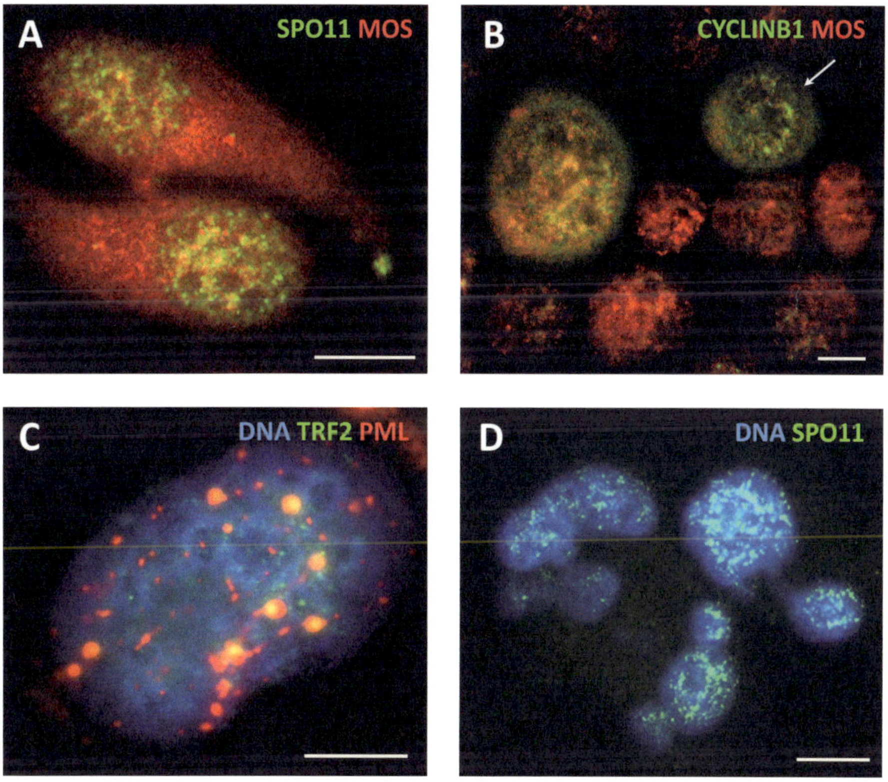

Figure 3.
Meiotic genes, alternative telomere lengthening, and mitotic slippage in B-RAF V600E and TP53-mutant melanoma SkMel28 cell line: (A) the expression of the meiotic MOS-kinase (sc-28,789) and recombination endonuclease SPO11 (sc-377,161) in cell nuclei of non-treated cells; (B) co-expression of MOS and cyclin B1 (sc-245) in rare polyploid cells and some metaphases [14] of nontreated control; (C) the polyploid cell on day 7 after doxorubicine treatment (500 nM for 24 h) maintains telomeres (marked by TRF2, 05-521, millipore) by alternative lengthening of telomeres (ALT) in promyelocytic leukemia (PML) (PA5-80910, thermo fisher scientific) bodies; and (D) two giant cells resistant to B-RAF inhibitor vemurafenib (50 nM for 24 h), with signs of mitotic slippage and multinucleation on day 21 after treatment show positivity for SPO11. Bars = 10 μm.

immunoglobulin gene diversification and class switch recombination, but mice lacking Spo11 had no detectable immune system defects [144]. SPO11 introduces meiotic recombination breaks in the chromosome DSB hotspots [145]. So, it is possible that senescence-associated DDR affecting the DSB hot spots (at least, in p53-nonfunctional tumors) can upregulate and attract SPO11. Localized clustered hotspots are a feature of meiotic recombination in *S. pombe*, mouse, and humans as well, but the factors that determine whether a given DNA sequence will be a DSB hotspot are not well understood in any organism. Such hotspots may appear due to underreplication of DNA in the heterochromatin, particularly in telomeres, e.g., in the drug-induced senescence of tumor cells [146]. Depletion of the H3K9me3 chromatin repressive hallmarks seems rather decisive for attraction of SPO11 to the hot spots [147]. This data shows that execution of the very definitive molecular biochemical mechanism of SPO11 is dependent on the permissive epigenetic chromatin organization of the very general character. Therefore, it is interesting to highlight the breaking through report showing the reset of senescence and abrogation of invasive growth achieved in melanoma by inhibition of the DNA demethylases [26].

Spo11 is the catalytic center of the meiotic recombination initiation mechanism, but it is not sufficient to generate DSBs: numerous additional proteins are also required; the main of them is Mre11-Rad50-Xrs2 (MRX). These proteins form a complex with multiple roles in many different aspects of DNA metabolism, including DNA repair, telomere maintenance, and checkpoint signaling. Mutant MRX complex leaves SPO11 accumulated to telomere ends with the nonreleased terminal chiasmata [148]. Although the SPO11 catalytic gene part is conserved, the proteins involved in meiotic recombination are generally among the more rapidly evolving of all cellular proteins: major challenges for them represent the whole genome duplications (WGDs) and the difficulties of auto- and allo-polyploids in the meiotic reduction divisions [149, 150].

The meiosis-specific histone methyltransferase gene PRDM9 has also been reported to be activated in melanoma alongside with other cancers, like embryonal carcinoma, astrocytoma, leukemia, colon, prostate, breast, and ovary cancers [151].

Another meiosis-specific gene involved in SPO11-mediated recombination regulation, TEX15, has been reported to be overexpressed in melanoma and other cancers including bladder, head and neck, and lung carcinomas, neuroblastomas, prostate tumors, and sarcomas [152].

The synapsis of homologous chromosomes in conventional meiotic prophase is marked by synaptonemal complex (SC). SC is a large zipper-like protein complex that connects one pair of sister chromatids to the homologous pair, so stabilizing the tetrad and ensuring proper homolog pairing. SC formation starts with the formation of axial element that consists from SC proteins 2 and 3 (SCP2 and SCP3). Then, the axial elements (at this point referred lateral elements) are joined by the transverse filaments formed by the SC protein 1 (SCP1) [153–155]. The central elements consists of SC central element 1 and 2 (encoded by SYCE1 and SYCE2) [156]. Notably, SYCP1 and SYCP3 genes both have been implicated in cancer. Both mRNA are expressed in a variety of cancers and cancer cell lines including melanoma [30, 31, 157, 158]. Moreover, SCP3 protein expression correlated with activated AKT (pAKT) signaling [159]. Overexpression of SCP3 was shown prognostically unfavorable for lung cancer [160].

HORMA domain containing 1 (Hormad1) is another protein associated with SC axis. It has multiple roles, but in general it coordinates DSB formation with synapsis and the timely progression of DSB repair through HR [161]. Hormad1 is significantly upregulated in several cancers and noted also in melanoma [37, 162]. Although the mechanism of its reactivation remains elusive, hypomethylation of the HORMAD1 promoter region correlates with its increased expression in breast cancer and small cell lung cancer [163, 164], suggesting at least partial involvement of epigenetic pathways.

Chromosome regulation in meiosis and in mitosis is dependent upon the cohesin complex. In mitotically dividing cells, this complex serves to hold sister chromatids until they settle in metaphase plate, becoming separated in anaphase while in conventional meiosis, sisters stay together through the whole meiosis I to ensure sister centromeres orientate to the same pole to drive the reductional segregation of bi-chromatid homologs. Although the structure of cohesin complexes involved in mitosis and meiosis is similar, the difference lies in subunit composition. In meiosis, specific paralogues of some of the cohesin proteins replace their mitotic counterparts [165]. One of the more prominent cohesin subunits that appears to be restricted to meiosis is REC8 (paralogous counterparts to the RAD21 mitotic cohesin) [165]. The upregulated expression of Rec8 protein was demonstrated in melanoma [37, 166] as well as in CTCL [139, 167], irradiated TP53-mutant lymphoma cell lines, HeLa, and breast and colon cancer cell lines [31, 168]. Recently it has been shown that REC8 imposed monopolarity of sister centromeres in mitotically dividing cells could result in uniparent disomy (UPD) at least in the model organism *S. pombe* (fission yeast) [169] possessing a facultative sex. REC8 in cooperation with *Mos*-kinase forms a monopolar spindle of octoploid lymphoma cells (after ionizing irradiation) which undergo recombination of DNA DSBs by meiotic recombinase DMC1 [62]. Interestingly, Rec8 does not appear to be incorporated into mitotic cohesin complex in HEK293 cells unless another meiosis-specific cohesin subunit, STAG3, is activated [170]. In melanoma, STAG3 as well as STAG2 (mitosis specific cohesin subunit) levels have been linked to the resistance of B-RAF inhibitors [171]. STAG cohesins also participate with CTCF in the topological suppression of transcription and it is the the reduced level of STAG3 that is associated with resistance to B-RAF inhibitors.

The cohesin-related regulators, SGO1/2 are also the meiosis-specific proteins that protect cohesin complex, in particular Rec8, from the protease separase-mediated cleavage at the centromeres of sister chromatids in meiosis I and retained Rec8 around the centromere until the start of anaphase II [172–174]. Upregulation of SGO2 expression has been demonstrated in melanoma [37] alongside with upregulation also in CTCL [139, 167] and SGO 1/2, along with REC8, in irradiated lymphoma cells [168]. However, the role of meiotic cohesins in cancer has not been extensively investigated.

Another meiosis-specific cohesin subunit, which has gene expression tightly restricted to the testis in healthy humans, is RAD21L (also RAD21/REC8 paralogue) [165]. However, it is also important for the maintenance of female fertility during natural aging [175].

While the majority of somatic cells are deficient in active telomerase, cancer cells not only can reactivate telomerase, but can also initiate a mechanism of the alternative telomere maintenance (ALT) in the absence of telomerase activity [176] or undergo transient ALT [177]. Some meiosis genes were found associated with supposed homology search in ALT [178, 179]. ALT requires a recombination-like mechanism to recognize the telomere end as DSBs and mediate the strand invasion of the end into a nonhomologous chromosome end. This strand invasion permits the initiation of a break-induced DNA replication process where the invaded non-homolog telomeric DNA serves as a replicative template for the invading telomere to elongate [180]. In summary, the review of the classic meiotic genes demonstrates their involvement in cancer, and melanoma in particular, although their function in cancer is ill defined.

6. Brainstorming session

> *"Nothing in biology makes sense except in the light of evolution"—Dobzhansky 1973 [181].*

B-RAF-mutant melanoma activates MEK-ERK proliferative pathway but cancer can be explained neither only by enhanced proliferation nor it can be reduced to somatic mutation theory, which has been shaken by cancer genome sequencing projects. Cancer is more complex than that [182]. B-RAF-and N-RAS-mutant nevi remaining quiescent and benign just support this notion. A very important role of OIS-induced cellular senescence for initiation of malignant tumors discovered by Serrano et al. [19] and the role of its epigenetic landscape have been revealed in recent years. Melanoma is interesting therefore as RAS, B-RAF mutations just produce this senescent background, which can undergo reverse by reprogramming resulting in drug resistance [25], but senescence can be again restored in invasive B-RAF-mutant melanoma by structurally unrelated silencing with H3K9 demethylases [26]. Thus, OIS senescence in cancer has a dynamic nature with the epigenetic component of the general character [183]. But melanoma is also interesting for the high overexpression of meiosis-related CT genes. Overexpression of CT antigens is prognostic for poor outcome of invasive melanoma; in addition, classic meiotic genes are known to be expressed in cancers [30, 31, 168] and also in melanoma [37]. Some authors reason that overlaying of meiotic protein aberrant activities over the normal mitotic cycle (termed "meiomitosis"), first of all of the stable cohesion of sister chromatids needed for meiosis I, is interfering with normal mitotic separation of chromatids, leading to aneuploidy, genome instability, and tumor progression [36, 37, 184, 185]. The questions arise: (1) whether the mitotic cycle in tumors is normal? (2) If the meiotic features found in tumors belong to conventional gametic meiosis? (3) If an aneuploidy can perpetuate the tumor growth? Let us begin with the latter. This problem is well known as "Aneuploidy Paradox" [186], which means that incorrect segregations of genetic material should hinder and prevent cell division; however, aneuploidy paradoxically is well known as correlating with tumor growth and aggression, which may be due to selection of the fittest aneuploid clones. This conundrum cannot be explained satisfactorily with clonal selection of rare positive mutations because the "Muller‘s Ratchet" [187] will inevitably accumulate deleterious mutation leading ultimately to extinction of the asexual cell line. The problem, of the "Muller Rachet", however is still explored by population evolutionists [188]. Aneuploidy in cancer arises from the inherent chromosome instability of polyploidy cells. So, we arrive here to the polyploidy which in different proportions is a very characteristic feature of all malignant tumors (comparing with their normal tissue origins), progresses with cancer aggression, and which up to now is often ignored by cancer researchers [189]. However, it is just a reversible polyploidy, which provides the extraordinary resistance of cancers to therapy [56, 190–192] and likely a cancer line immortality as such. Moreover, our studies brought us to the notion of a cancer life cycle, composed of a cell cycle (lasting 17-23 h) and ploidy cycle (reversible polyploidization which takes 1–2 weeks or more), both cycles are reciprocally linked [32, 193]. This reciprocal cancer life cycle is an analogue of the "neosis" of cancer cells, related to polyploidy and senescence with rejuvenation of reduced offsprings described by Rajaraman [194, 195] and was confirmed in tumors by multiple authors [190–192], also in melanoma [59]. Thus, the answer to the first question is that the cell cycle in cancers including melanoma is not conventional and at least, in the tumor subpopulation, it is composed of two reciprocally joined different cycles, conventional mitotic and a ploidy cycle, one being quick and another being slow. The latter is often overlooked [189] as being hidden due to the low proportion in relation to the mitotic cycles. The ploidy cycle of giant cells associated with senescence reprogramming becomes clearly manifested in resistant tumors after high dosage DNA damage with anticancer drugs and ionizing irradiation [177, 196–198]. Therefore, cancer research needs prolong follow up of individual cells and ploidy measurements [177, 191, 199, 200]. Tumor cells enter this ploidy cycle when they senesce by OIS or get the DNA damage in any other way (e.g., by ionizing irradiation or oxidative stress). If the treatment is harsh, the majority of induced giant cells will die in the time course, during mitotic catastrophe or in unsuccessful attempts of multipolar or aberrant bipolar bridged mitoses, but a minor minority of resistant cancer cells repair the DNA damage and repopulate tumors through depolyploidization by budding or other type of ploidy reduction [33, 56, 189, 191, 201, 202]. So, in our brainstorming session, we arrived to ploidy cycles and DNA damage. Here is a right link to the origin of meiosis and sex. The whole genome duplications (WGD) is a well-known driver of gene and species evolution [203] and appeared already in prokaryotes as the first evolutionary steps toward eukaryotic sex [204]. The most immediate reasons of the meiosis origin were the necessity to repair DNA damage [205]. Another reason, coupled to the first, was the relief of mutational load of aneuploidy resulting from polyploidy when it was advantageous to have more than one copy of the genome per cell [206]. Thus, the aneuploidy paradox in cancer might be resolved by asexual (somatic) meiosis (including recombination and reduction) and this meiosis is very likely ancestral. Briefly, the evolution of meiosis in eukaryotes could start from polyploid endomitosis (insect-type, without actual karyotomy), (enriched in MOS-kinase as found in tumor cells) [207], followed by zygotic meiosis, and ending in gametic meiosis in most extant vertebrates [149, 208–210]. Meiosis originated in evolution several times; there is also a view that individual blocks of genetic program of meiotic regulation could evolve independently [211]. Considering the expression of CT genes not only in testis but also in ovaria, early embryo and placenta, Loyd Old [212] associated their expression with the female gametogenesis-like program in tumor cells by formulating the title of his article "Cancer is a somatic cell pregnancy." Some researchers consider a possible parthenogenetic variant of the embryological in essence theory of cancer which is known from the nineteenth century [29, 213] while ontogenetic variant of this theory for the origin of tumors termed "a life-code" has been recently suggested by Jinsong Liu [214]. An interesting asexual parthenogenetic variant for triploid tumors, which are typical for resistant cancers may be achieved by digyny (69, XXY, in case of male cancers) [215]. Some observations suggest that triploidy may exchange with diploid subline on the basis of multinucleated giant cells in the same tumor [216]. The cycle of cancer stem cells likely can start with the relic uniparental disomy. The latter is described in facultative sex of the fission yeast [169], in plants, stressed and spontaneously [217] and in senescing human cells [218]. All these parasexual mechanisms may include aberrant meiotic elements and genes activity [62] and may exist in parallel or as a complex chain of one process of the survival support and escape of resistant tumors. In fact, their studies are only started. So, the answer to the second question if we should reckon exclusively with the mechanisms of conventional gametic meiosis in somatic tumors is also negative. SC in tumors was never found although the relevant genes and proteins ectopically expressed [62, 160], including melanoma [37]. We should rather reckon with evolutionary forms of meiosis in asexual life cycles. This turn of reasoning is becoming particularly context-updated if we also consider the recent gene expression phylostratigraphic analysis showing that ancestral regulatory networks drive cancer [219]. The latter in turn is associated with polyploidy [220]. Moreover, in recent time, the ancient inverted meiosis (IM) appeared on the stage [221]. IM does not require the cohesion of sister chromatids (thus, SC is not needed): the homologs are joined by their ends, recombine by sub-telomeric sequences, segregate sisters in the first meiosis and homologs in the second. Thus, IM can repair the damaged telomeres, provide some degree of genetic diversity, and not the least, it can count homologous chromosome pairs, to get rid of aneuploidy. Strikingly, IM was revealed in the proportion of normal human oocytes sorting out the aneuploid embryos in a polar body [222]. Although SC is not needed, however the telomere clustering at the spindle pole body for the chromosome homology search by spinning the chromosomes, for DNA recombination between homologs, is needed. Although currently the study of IM in human cancer is in infancy [62], the IM related to telomere DSBs well fits several peculiarities found in tumors: cellular senescence linked to telomere attrition, polyploidy associated with cellular senescence, mitotic slippage, reprogramming, and alternative telomere lengthening characteristic for some cancers [62]. We proposed a hypothesis that ALT-associated PML bodies in mitotic slippage of tumor cells may serve as a site for IM recombination repair [177]. Interestingly, the meiotic genes involved in the homology search and recombination RAD21L (Rec8 paralog) and Hop2-Mnd1 heterodimer (RAD51-dependent) were found associated with ALT [178, 179]. The expression of the proteins, which may be involved in IM-related ALT (SPO11, MOS, TRF2-colocalised with PML-bodies), and mitotic slippage were also observed in polyploidy cells of B-RAF V600E mutant melanoma SkMel28 cell line treated with doxorubicin and vemurafenib (mutated B-RAF-inhibitor) (**Figure 3**). The question how much the meiotic features in tumors are stochastic and how much program-directed is central for addressing the problem. The most prominent feature of cancer is adaptation to extinction by the mechanisms acquired in the evolution of life on earth. The naturally occurring tumors are found already in *Hydra* [223]. When the organisms were challenged by extinction, they have adapted to it by transient polyploidy, epigenetic plasticity, including pluripotent stemness with its bivalency of genes, intrinsically disordered proteins, and rearrangement of the nuclear architecture domains by phase transitions—these epigenetic adaptations are by two orders faster than the gene mutation-selection-based process would allow [224]. In accord, the expression of stemness genes, early stress response genes, epigenetic master activator CTCFL/BORIS and in particular, CT antigens genes as universal adaptors for reconstruction of the genome functional network—all these epigenetic evolutionary adaptations are found in melanoma, which are highly mortal-risky and treatment resistant in patients. At the same time, the tumor pathways are rare evolutionary attractors of the genome multi-dimensional network [225], entrapping cancer cells by the therapy resistance—only a small number of cells, but inevitably survive and repopulate the tumors [56, 177]. These rare genome space states can be only chosen by the mechanisms of nonequilibrium thermodynamics, which is by coherating fluctuations, through the method of trial and error [224, 226]. Those are inevitably accompanied by a lot of cell death and a lot of aberrant phenotypes, which may persist as transient or axillary to reproductive cancer cell line. The fidelity of the genome achieved through the evolutionary meiosis and ploidy life cycles can counteract the aneuploidy; otherwise, tumor cells may balance between both options. The snap-shot studies, not considering this factor (e.g., the productive expression of meiotic genes in only sub-population of tumor cells) can thus bring to misleading interpretations [227]. Moreover, both forward and reverse mutations occurring by gene conversion were recently found in the oldest (from 1951) human cancer cell line cervical carcinoma HeLa [228], which is also known serving a positive control for the meiotic proteins antibodies and expresses them in reversible polyploidy cycles [31]. As suggested by Maciver in 2016 [229], gene conversion in asexual polyploid species can compensate the "Muller's Ratchet." Gene conversion is the process by which one DNA sequence replaces a homologous sequence such that the sequences become identical after the conversion event. In this case, the nonreciprocal "copy-paste" recombination is occurring which is stimulated by

DNA strand breaks in hot spots [230]. This type of the genetic reconstruction seems also to be compatible with tumor cell senescence, mitotic slippage, and ALT.

7. Conclusion

The CT antigens and meiotic genes enhanced expression in tumors, including B-RAF-mutant melanoma, is associated with poor prognosis for the patient survival and treatment outcomes. The review shows that the functions of CTA and meiotic genes in cancer are multilayered: they involve genetic, whole-genomic, cytogenetic, epigenomic, and posttranslational levels of regulation, which are evolutionarily evolved. That means that the expression of CT antigens and meiotic genes is in general adaptive, explaining the correlation of this expression with poor melanoma prognosis. The matter concerns some recently acknowledged biological processes, whose mechanisms and thermodynamics are not fully understood. These are reversible polyploidy and reversible senescence, transient ALT, gene conversion, and likely also several forms of evolutionary, nonconventional, asexual meiosis and parthenogenesis. The fidelity of the genome aimed through the evolutionary meiosis and ploidy life cycles can potentially compensate the aneuploidy, or the tumor cells may balance between the advantages and disadvantages of both options [150]. All these questions still remain open for future studies.

Acknowledgements

The authors thank Olga Anatskaya (St. Petersburg) for advice in bioinformatic methodology and Madara Kreismane for technical support for manuscript preparation.

This work was supported by a grant from the European Regional Development Fund (ERDF) projects No. 1.1.1.1/18/A/099, 1.1.1.2/VIAA/3/19/463 for K.S. and Student Scholarship from the University of Latvia Foundation to N.M.V.

Conflict of interest

The authors declare no conflict of interest.

Appendix A

Gene	Symbol	Log2FC
Melanoma-associated antigen 3	MAGEA3	7.645235
Melanoma-associated antigen 12	MAGEA12	7.348702
Cancer/testis antigen 2	CTAG2	7.111641
MAGE family member C2	MAGEC2	6.874003
Melanoma-associated antigen 6	MAGEA6	6.828297
Chondrosarcoma-associated Gene 1	CSAG1	6.204377
Preferentially expressed antigen of melanoma	PRAME	5.821726
Melanoma-associated antigen 1	MAGEA1	5.752684
MAGE family member A2B	MAGEA2B	5.738676

Gene	Symbol	Log2FC
Melanoma-associated antigen 4	MAGEA4	5.327805
Prostate-associated gene protein 5	PAGE5	5.246215
Prostate-associated gene protein 2	PAGE2	4.905513
MAGE family member B2	MAGEB2	4.803597
Melanoma-associated antigen 11	MAGEA11	3.985815
PAGE family member 2B	PAGE2B	3.714482
MAGE family member C1	MAGEC1	3.522569
Melanoma-associated antigen 10	MAGEA10	3.168079
Cancer/testis antigen family 25, member 1a	DSCR8	2.770747
Interleukin 13 receptor subunit alpha 2	IL13RA2	2.338307
Transgelin	TAGLN	2.28783
Catenin alpha 2	CTNNA2	2.112868
Mesenteric estrogen-dependent adipogenesis	MEDAG	2.087961
PDZ binding kinase	PBK	2.022606
Homeobox protein BarH-like 1	BARX1	1.99113
Centrosomal protein 55	CEP55	1.86278
Sperm-associated antigen 4	SPAG4	1.521662
T-cell activation RhoGTPase activating protein	TAGAP	1.510325
MAGE family member B17	MAGEB17	1.498956
Homeobox protein ARX	ARX	1.147917
Outer dense fiber of sperm tails 3B	ODF3B	1.144663
ATPase family AAA domain containing 2	ATAD2	1.116308
MAGE family member D1	MAGED1	0.941916
GATA zinc finger domain containing 2A	GATAD2A	0.892566
ADAM metallopeptidase domain 28	ADAM28	0.838868
Phosphotyrosine picked threonine-protein kinase	TTK	0.78873
Opa-interacting protein 5	OIP5	0.775664
Acrosin binding protein	ACRBP	0.518623
Nucleolar protein 4 like	NOL4L	0.487608
GATA zinc finger domain containing 2B	GATAD2B	0.484958
Outer dense fiber of sperm tails 2	ODF2	0.40552
MAGE family member F1	MAGEF1	0.334573
Cancer/testis antigen 101	KIAA0100	0.315249
Transgelin 2	TAGLN2	0.241303
DDB1- and CUL4-associated factor 12	DCAF12	0.228037

Appendix Table 1.
The list of genes with significantly upregulated expression of CT antigenes in the cohort of 51 primary melanomas compared to 27 B-RAF V600E-mutant nevi from the NCBI's Gene Expression Omnibus GSE98394 dataset (described in detail in [80]). EdgeR [127] was used to perform differential expression analysis through the generalized linear model approach. The differentially upregulated in melanoma genes (log2FC > 0, p < 0.01) were filtered for CT antigenes. The whole CT antigenes list comprising of 220 genes was acquired from the CT database [70]. Expression is presented as log_2 FC units.

Gene	Symbol	Log2FC
SPANX family member A2	SPANXA2	4.748924
SPANX family member B1	SPANXB1	4.617090
Sperm protein associated with the nucleus, X-linked, family member A1	SPANXA1	4.501381
Transgelin 3	TAGLN3	4.426952
SPANX family member D	SPANXD	3.947176
Transmembrane protein with EGF-like and two follistatin-like domains 2	TMEFF2	3.767568
SPANX family member C	SPANXC	3.684016
Interleukin 13 receptor subunit alpha 2	IL13RA2	2.558249
Coiled-coil domain containing 33	CCDC33	2.399770
PAGE family member 4	PAGE4	2.248496
Nucleolar protein 4	NOL4	2.078128
Tudor domain containing 15	TDRD15	1.896378
VENT homeobox pseudogene 1	VENTXP1	1.859120
DDB1 and CUL4 associated factor 12 like 2	DCAF12L2	1.816185
SPANXA2 overlapping transcript 1	SPANXA2-OT1	1.793161
RNA binding motif protein 46	RBM46	1.765131
F-box protein 39	FBXO39	1.599419
ADAM metallopeptidase domain 28	ADAM28	1.545184
T cell activation RhoGTPase activating protein	TAGAP	1.530934
Tektin 5	TEKT5	1.443142
Maelstrom spermatogenic transposon silencer	MAEL	1.415596
Actin-like 8	ACTL8	1.358688
MAGE family member A1	MAGEA1	1.315031
ADAM metallopeptidase domain 21	ADAM21	1.210916
PRAME N-terminal-like, pseudogene	PRAMENP	1.202568
MAGE family member A10	MAGEA10	1.163532
MAGEA10-MAGEA5 readthrough	MAGEA10-MAGEA5	1.163181
NLR family pyrin domain containing 4	NLRP4	1.053507
ADAM metallopeptidase domain 22	ADAM22	0.922948
Acrosin binding protein	ACRBP	0.854224
Transmembrane protein 108	TMEM108	0.793037
Ankyrin repeat domain 45	ANKRD45	0.779239
BAGE family member 2	BAGE2	0.733106
Mesenteric estrogen dependent adipogenesis	MEDAG	0.72858
Sperm associated antigen 4	SPAG4	0.70602

Gene	Symbol	Log2FC
Placenta enriched 1	PLAC1	0.669653
Fetal and adult testis expressed 1	FATE1	0.61294
Transmembrane protein with EGF-like and two follistatin-like domains 1	TMEFF1	0.603075
Piwi-like RNA-mediated gene silencing 4	PIWIL4	0.601545
Piwi-like RNA-mediated gene silencing 2	PIWIL2	0.566213
Centrosomal protein 290	CEP290	0.489041
Stromal antigen 2	STAG2	0.470227
Cutaneous T cell lymphoma-associated antigen 1	CTAGE1	0.457364
SSX family member 2 interacting protein	SSX2IP	0.426617
Transgelin	TAGLN	0.425961
MSANTD3-TMEFF1 readthrough	MSANTD3-TMEFF1	0.423834
Tudor domain containing	TDRD6	0.344416
ATPase family AAA domain containing 2	ATAD2	0.322527
TTK protein kinase	TTK	0.316241
ATPase family AAA domain containing 2B	ATAD2B	0.30301
Stromal antigen 1	STAG1	0.277385
OIP5 antisense RNA 1	OIP5-AS1	0.26571
M-phase phosphoprotein 10	MPHOSPH10	0.235959
DDB1- and CUL4-associated factor 12	DCAF12	0.158102

Appendix Table 2.
Significantly upregulated expression of CT antigenes in the cohort of 368 melanoma metastases compared to 103 primary melanomas from the TCGA-SKCM dataset (https://www.cancer.gov/tcga). The data was extracted from the TCGA database using the TCGA Biolinks Bioconductor package [124]. EdgeR [127] was used to perform differential expression analysis through the generalized linear model approach and the differentially expressed genes (DEGs) which were upregulated in metastatic melanoma (log2FC > 0, $p < 0.01$) were filtered for CT antigens. The CT antigenes list comprising of 220 genes was acquired from the CT database [70]. Expression is presented as log_2FC units.

Author details

Dace Pjanova[1*], Ninel M. Vainshelbaum[1,2], Kristine Salmina[1] and Jekaterina Erenpreisa[1,2]

1 Latvian Biomedical Research and Study Centre, Riga, Latvia

2 Faculty of Biology, University of Latvia, Riga, Latvia

*Address all correspondence to: dace@biomed.lu.lv

References

[1] Network TCGA. Genomic classification of cutaneous melanoma. Cell. 2015;**161**(7):1681-1696. DOI: 10.1016/j.cell.2015.05.044

[2] Ascierto PA, Kirkwood JM, Grob JJ, Simeone E, Grimaldi AM, Maio M, et al. The role of BRAF V600 mutation in melanoma. Journal of Translational Medicine. 2012;**10**:85. DOI: 10.1186/1479-5876-10-85

[3] McCubrey JA, Steelman LS, Chappell WH, Abrams SL, Wong EW, Chang F, et al. Roles of the Raf/MEK/ERK pathway in cell growth, malignant transformation and drug resistance. Biochimica et Biophysica Acta. 2007;**1773**(8):1263-1284. DOI: 10.1016/j.bbamcr.2006.10.001

[4] Flaherty KT, Puzanov I, Kim KB, Ribas A, McArthur GA, Sosman JA, et al. Inhibition of mutated, activated BRAF in metastatic melanoma. The New England Journal of Medicine. 2010;**363**(9):809-819. DOI: 10.1056/NEJMoa1002011

[5] Flaherty KT, Robert C, Hersey P, Nathan P, Garbe C, Milhem M, et al. Improved survival with MEK inhibition in BRAF-mutated melanoma. The New England Journal of Medicine. 2012;**367**(2):107-114. DOI: 10.1056/NEJMoa1203421

[6] Long GV, Stroyakovskiy D, Gogas H, Levchenko E, de Braud F, Larkin J, et al. Dabrafenib and trametinib versus dabrafenib and placebo for Val600 BRAF-mutant melanoma: A multicentre, double-blind, phase 3 randomised controlled trial. Lancet (London, England). 2015;**386**(9992):444-451. DOI: 10.1016/s0140-6736(15)60898-4

[7] Chapman PB, Hauschild A, Robert C, Haanen JB, Ascierto P, Larkin J, et al. Improved survival with vemurafenib in melanoma with BRAF V600E mutation. The New England Journal of Medicine. 2011;**364**(26):2507-2516. DOI: 10.1056/NEJMoa1103782

[8] Falchook GS, Long GV, Kurzrock R, Kim KB, Arkenau TH, Brown MP, et al. Dabrafenib in patients with melanoma, untreated brain metastases, and other solid tumours: A phase 1 dose-escalation trial. Lancet (London, England). 2012;**379**(9829):1893-1901. DOI: 10.1016/s0140-6736(12)60398-5

[9] Hauschild A, Grob JJ, Demidov LV, Jouary T, Gutzmer R, Millward M, et al. Dabrafenib in BRAF-mutated metastatic melanoma: A multicentre, open-label, phase 3 randomised controlled trial. Lancet (London, England). 2012;**380**(9839):358-365. DOI: 10.1016/s0140-6736(12)60868-x

[10] Sosman JA, Kim KB, Schuchter L, Gonzalez R, Pavlick AC, Weber JS, et al. Survival in BRAF V600-mutant advanced melanoma treated with vemurafenib. The New England Journal of Medicine. 2012;**366**(8):707-714. DOI: 10.1056/NEJMoa1112302

[11] Johnson DB, Sosman JA. Therapeutic advances and treatment options in metastatic melanoma. JAMA Oncology. 2015;**1**(3):380-386. DOI: 10.1001/jamaoncol.2015.0565

[12] Ascierto PA, McArthur GA, Dréno B, Atkinson V, Liszkay G, Di Giacomo AM, et al. Cobimetinib combined with vemurafenib in advanced BRAF(V600)-mutant melanoma (coBRIM): Updated efficacy results from a randomised, double-blind, phase 3 trial. The Lancet Oncology. 2016;**17**(9):1248-1260. DOI: 10.1016/s1470-2045(16)30122-x

[13] Pollock PM, Harper UL, Hansen KS, Yudt LM, Stark M, Robbins CM, et al. High frequency of BRAF mutations in

nevi. Nature Genetics. 2003;**33**(1):19-20. DOI: 10.1038/ng1054

[14] Davies H, Bignell GR, Cox C, Stephens P, Edkins S, Clegg S, et al. Mutations of the BRAF gene in human cancer. Nature. 2002;**417**(6892):949-954. DOI: 10.1038/nature00766

[15] Michaloglou C, Vredeveld LC, Soengas MS, Denoyelle C, Kuilman T, van der Horst CM, et al. BRAFE600-associated senescence-like cell cycle arrest of human naevi. Nature. 2005;**436**(7051):720-724. DOI: 10.1038/nature03890

[16] Bevona C, Goggins W, Quinn T, Fullerton J, Tsao H. Cutaneous melanomas associated with nevi. Archives of Dermatology. 2003;**139**(12):1620-1624; discussion 1624. DOI: 10.1001/archderm.139.12.1620

[17] Collado M, Gil J, Efeyan A, Guerra C, Schuhmacher AJ, Barradas M, et al. Tumour biology: Senescence in premalignant tumours. Nature. 2005;**436**(7051):642. DOI: 10.1038/436642a

[18] Chen Z, Trotman LC, Shaffer D, Lin HK, Dotan ZA, Niki M, et al. Crucial role of p53-dependent cellular senescence in suppression of Pten-deficient tumorigenesis. Nature. 2005;**436**(7051):725-730. DOI: 10.1038/nature03918

[19] Serrano M, Lin AW, McCurrach ME, Beach D, Lowe SW. Oncogenic ras provokes premature cell senescence associated with accumulation of p53 and p16INK4a. Cell. 1997;**88**(5):593-602. DOI: 10.1016/s0092-8674(00)81902-9

[20] Collado M, Blasco MA, Serrano M. Cellular senescence in cancer and aging. Cell. 2007;**130**(2):223-233. DOI: 10.1016/j.cell.2007.07.003

[21] Sabisz M, Skladanowski A. Cancer stem cells and escape from drug-induced premature senescence in human lung tumor cells: Implications for drug resistance and in vitro drug screening models. Cell Cycle (Georgetown, Texas). 2009;**8**(19):3208-3217. DOI: 10.4161/cc.8.19.9758

[22] Angelini PD, Zacarias Fluck MF, Pedersen K, Parra-Palau JL, Guiu M, Bernadó Morales C, et al. Constitutive HER2 signaling promotes breast cancer metastasis through cellular senescence. Cancer Research. 2013;**73**(1):450-458. DOI: 10.1158/0008-5472.can-12-2301

[23] Campisi J. Aging, cellular senescence, and cancer. Annual Review of Physiology. 2013;**75**:685-705. DOI: 10.1146/annurev-physiol-030212-183653

[24] Erenpreisa J, Salmina K, Cragg MS. Accelerated senescence of cancer stem cells: A failure to thrive or a route to survival? In: Dorszewska J, Kozubski W, editors. Senescence—Physiology or Pathology. London UK: IntechOpen; 2017. p. 18. DOI: 10.5772/intechopen.68582.

[25] Milanovic M, Fan DNY, Belenki D, Däbritz JHM, Zhao Z, Yu Y, et al. Senescence-associated reprogramming promotes cancer stemness. Nature. 2018;**553**(7686):96-100. DOI: 10.1038/nature25167

[26] Yu Y, Schleich K, Yue B, Ji S, Lohneis P, Kemper K, et al. Targeting the senescence-overriding cooperative activity of structurally unrelated H3K9 demethylases in melanoma. Cancer Cell. 2018;**33**(2):322-336.e328. DOI: 10.1016/j.ccell.2018.01.002

[27] Chadee DN. Involvement of mixed lineage kinase 3 in cancer. Canadian Journal of Physiology and Pharmacology. 2013;**91**(4):268-274. DOI: 10.1139/cjpp-2012-0258

[28] Kleckner N. Meiosis: How could it work? Proceedings of the National Academy of Sciences of the United

States of America. 1996;**93**(16):8167-8174. DOI: 10.1073/pnas.93.16.8167

[29] Erenpreiss JO. Current Concepts of Malignant Growth. Part a. from a Normal Cell to Cancer. Riga: Zvaigzne; 1993

[30] Kalejs M, Ivanov A, Plakhins G, Cragg MS, Emzinsh D, Illidge TM, et al. Upregulation of meiosis-specific genes in lymphoma cell lines following genotoxic insult and induction of mitotic catastrophe. BMC Cancer. 2006;**6**:6. DOI: 10.1186/1471-2407-6-6

[31] Ianzini F, Kosmacek EA, Nelson ES, Napoli E, Erenpreisa J, Kalejs M, et al. Activation of meiosis-specific genes is associated with depolyploidization of human tumor cells following radiation-induced mitotic catastrophe. Cancer Research. 2009;**69**(6):2296-2304. DOI: 10.1158/0008-5472.can-08-3364

[32] Erenpreisa J, Cragg MS. MOS, aneuploidy and the ploidy cycle of cancer cells. Oncogene. 2010;**29**(40):5447-5451. DOI: 10.1038/onc.2010.310

[33] Erenpreisa J, Cragg MS. Three steps to the immortality of cancer cells: Senescence, polyploidy and self-renewal. Cancer Cell International. 2013;**13**(1):92. DOI: 10.1186/1475-2867-13-92

[34] Nielsen AY, Gjerstorff MF. Ectopic expression of testis germ cell proteins in cancer and its potential role in genomic instability. International Journal of Molecular Sciences. 2016;**17**(6):890. DOI: 10.3390/ijms17060890

[35] Feichtinger J, McFarlane RJ. Meiotic gene activation in somatic and germ cell tumours. Andrology. 2019;7(4):415-427. DOI: 10.1111/andr.12628

[36] Gantchev J, Martínez Villarreal A, Gunn S, Zetka M, Ødum N, Litvinov IV. The ectopic expression of meiCT genes promotes meiomitosis and may facilitate carcinogenesis. Cell Cycle (Georgetown, Texas). 2020;**19**(8):837-854. DOI: 10.1080/15384101.2020.1743902

[37] Lindsey SF, Byrnes DM, Eller MS, Rosa AM, Dabas N, Escandon J, et al. Potential role of meiosis proteins in melanoma chromosomal instability. Journal of Skin Cancer. 2013;**2013**:190109. DOI: 10.1155/2013/190109

[38] Rodier F, Coppé JP, Patil CK, Hoeijmakers WA, Muñoz DP, Raza SR, et al. Persistent DNA damage signalling triggers senescence-associated inflammatory cytokine secretion. Nature Cell Biology. 2009;**11**(8):973-979. DOI: 10.1038/ncb1909

[39] Aylon Y, Oren M. p53: Guardian of ploidy. Molecular Oncology. 2011;**5**(4):315-323. DOI: 10.1016/j.molonc.2011.07.007

[40] Kastan MB, Onyekwere O, Sidransky D, Vogelstein B, Craig RW. Participation of p53 protein in the cellular response to DNA damage. Cancer Research. 1991;**51**(23 Pt 1):6304-6311

[41] Baryshev M, Inashkina I, Salmina K, Huna A, Jackson TR, Erenpreisa J. DNA methylation of the Oct4A enhancers in embryonal carcinoma cells after etoposide treatment is associated with alternative splicing and altered pluripotency in reversibly senescent cells. Cell Cycle (Georgetown, Texas). 2018;**17**(3):362-366. DOI: 10.1080/15384101.2018.1426412

[42] Olivier M, Hollstein M, Hainaut P. TP53 mutations in human cancers: Origins, consequences, and clinical use. Cold Spring Harbor Perspectives in Biology. 2010;**2**(1):a001008. DOI: 10.1101/cshperspect.a001008

[43] Kastan MB. Wild-type p53: Tumors can't stand it. Cell. 2007;**128**(5):837-840. DOI: 10.1016/j.cell.2007.02.022

[44] Kastenhuber ER, Lowe SW. Putting p53 in context. Cell. 2017;**170**(6):1062-1078. DOI: 10.1016/j.cell.2017.08.028

[45] Hocker T, Tsao H. Ultraviolet radiation and melanoma: A systematic review and analysis of reported sequence variants. Human Mutation. 2007;**28**(6):578-588. DOI: 10.1002/humu.20481

[46] Box NF, Vukmer TO, Terzian T. Targeting p53 in melanoma. Pigment Cell & Melanoma Research. 2014;**27**(1):8-10. DOI: 10.1111/pcmr.12180

[47] Potrony M, Badenas C, Aguilera P, Puig-Butille JA, Carrera C, Malvehy J, et al. Update in genetic susceptibility in melanoma. Annals of Translational Medicine. 2015;**3**(15):210. DOI: 10.3978/j.issn.2305-5839.2015.08.11

[48] Stott FJ, Bates S, James MC, McConnell BB, Starborg M, Brookes S, et al. The alternative product from the human CDKN2A locus, p14(ARF), participates in a regulatory feedback loop with p53 and MDM2. The EMBO Journal. 1998;**17**(17):5001-5014. DOI: 10.1093/emboj/17.17.5001

[49] Patton EE, Widlund HR, Kutok JL, Kopani KR, Amatruda JF, Murphey RD, et al. BRAF mutations are sufficient to promote nevi formation and cooperate with p53 in the genesis of melanoma. Current Biology: CB. 2005;**15**(3):249-254. DOI: 10.1016/j.cub.2005.01.031

[50] Vredeveld LC, Possik PA, Smit MA, Meissl K, Michaloglou C, Horlings HM, et al. Abrogation of BRAFV600E-induced senescence by PI3K pathway activation contributes to melanomagenesis. Genes & Development. 2012;**26**(10):1055-1069. DOI: 10.1101/gad.187252.112

[51] Ziegler CGK, Allon SJ, Nyquist SK, Mbano IM, Miao VN, Tzouanas CN, et al. SARS-CoV-2 receptor ACE2 is an interferon-stimulated gene in human airway epithelial cells and is detected in specific cell subsets across tissues. Cell. 2020;**181**(5):1016-1035 e1019. DOI: 10.1016/j.cell.2020.04.035

[52] Riffell JL, Zimmerman C, Khong A, McHardy LM, Roberge M. Effects of chemical manipulation of mitotic arrest and slippage on cancer cell survival and proliferation. Cell Cycle (Georgetown, Texas). 2009;**8**(18):3025-3038

[53] Zhang S, Mercado-Uribe I, Xing Z, Sun B, Kuang J, Liu J. Generation of cancer stem-like cells through the formation of polyploid giant cancer cells. Oncogene. 2014;**33**(1):116-128. DOI: 10.1038/onc.2013.96

[54] Mosieniak G, Sliwinska MA, Alster O, Strzeszewska A, Sunderland P, Piechota M, et al. Polyploidy formation in doxorubicin-treated cancer cells can favor escape from senescence. Neoplasia (New York, NY). 2015;**17**(12):882-893. DOI: 10.1016/j.neo.2015.11.008

[55] Erenpreisa J, Salmiņa K, Belyayev A, Inashkina I, Cragg MS. Survival at the brink. In: Hayat MA, editor. Autophagy: Cancer, Other Pathologies, Inflammation, Immunity, Infection, and Aging. Vol. 3. 1 ed. Amsterdam, The Netherlands: Elsevier; 2017. pp. 275-294

[56] Illidge TM, Cragg MS, Fringes B, Olive P, Erenpreisa JA. Polyploid giant cells provide a survival mechanism for p53 mutant cells after DNA damage. Cell Biology International. 2000;**24**(9):621-633. DOI: 10.1006/cbir.2000.0557

[57] Shaffer SM, Dunagin MC, Torborg SR, Torre EA, Emert B, Krepler C, et al. Rare cell variability and drug-induced reprogramming as a mode of cancer drug resistance. Nature. 2017;**546**(7658):431-435. DOI: 10.1038/nature22794

[58] Vilgelm AE, Cobb P, Malikayil K, Flaherty D, Andrew Johnson C,

Raman D, et al. MDM2 antagonists counteract drug-induced DNA damage. eBioMedicine. 2017;**24**:43-55. DOI: 10.1016/j.ebiom.2017.09.016

[59] Leikam C, Hufnagel AL, Otto C, Murphy DJ, Mühling B, Kneitz S, et al. In vitro evidence for senescent multinucleated melanocytes as a source for tumor-initiating cells. Cell Death & Disease. 2015;**6**(4):e1711. DOI: 10.1038/cddis.2015.71

[60] Sagata N. What does Mos do in oocytes and somatic cells? BioEssays. 1997;**19**(1):13-21. DOI: 10.1002/bies.950190105

[61] Tachibana K, Tanaka D, Isobe T, Kishimoto T. c-Mos forces the mitotic cell cycle to undergo meiosis II to produce haploid gametes. Proceedings of the National Academy of Sciences of the United States of America. 2000;**97**(26):14301-14306. DOI: 10.1073/pnas.97.26.14301

[62] Salmina K, Huna A, Kalejs M, Pjanova D, Scherthan H, Cragg MS, et al. The cancer aneuploidy paradox: In the light of evolution. Genes. 2019;**10**(2):83. DOI: 10.3390/genes10020083

[63] Bruggen PVD, Szikora J-P, Boël P, Wildmann C, Somville M, Sensi M, et al. Autologous cytolytic T lymphocytes recognize a MAGE-1 nonapeptide on melanomas expressing HLA-Cw* 1601. European Journal of Immunology. 1994;**24**(9):2134-2140. DOI: 10.1002/eji.1830240930

[64] Boël P, Wildmann C, Sensi ML, Brasseur R, Renauld JC, Coulie P, et al. BAGE: A new gene encoding an antigen recognized on human melanomas by cytolytic T lymphocytes. Immunity. 1995;**2**(2):167-175. DOI: 10.1016/s1074-7613(95)80053-0

[65] Chen YT, Güre AO, Tsang S, Stockert E, Jäger E, Knuth A, et al. Identification of multiple cancer/testis antigens by allogeneic antibody screening of a melanoma cell line library. Proceedings of the National Academy of Sciences of the United States of America. 1998;**95**(12):6919-6923. DOI: 10.1073/pnas.95.12.6919

[66] Bruggen P, Traversari C, Chomez P, Lurquin C, De Plaen E, Van den Eynde B, et al. A gene encoding an antigen recognized by cytolytic T lymphocytes on a human melanoma. Science (New York, N.Y.). 1991;**254**(5038):1643-1647. DOI: 10.1126/science.1840703

[67] Van den Eynde B, Peeters O, De Backer O, Gaugler B, Lucas S, Boon T. A new family of genes coding for an antigen recognized by autologous cytolytic T lymphocytes on a human melanoma. The Journal of Experimental Medicine. 1995;**182**(3):689-698. DOI: 10.1084/jem.182.3.689

[68] Gaugler B, Van den Eynde B, van der Bruggen P, Romero P, Gaforio JJ, De Plaen E, et al. Human gene MAGE-3 codes for an antigen recognized on a melanoma by autologous cytolytic T lymphocytes. The Journal of Experimental Medicine. 1994;**179**(3):921-930. DOI: 10.1084/jem.179.3.921

[69] De Backer O, Arden KC, Boretti M, Vantomme V, De Smet C, Czekay S, et al. Characterization of the GAGE genes that are expressed in various human cancers and in normal testis. Cancer Research. 1999;**59**(13):3157-3165

[70] Sahin U, Türeci O, Schmitt H, Cochlovius B, Johannes T, Schmits R, et al. Human neoplasms elicit multiple specific immune responses in the autologous host. Proceedings of the National Academy of Sciences of the United States of America. 1995;**92**(25):11810-11813. DOI: 10.1073/pnas.92.25.11810

[71] Almeida LG, Sakabe NJ, deOliveira AR, Silva MC,

Mundstein AS, Cohen T, et al. CT database: A knowledge-base of high-throughput and curated data on cancer-testis antigens. Nucleic Acids Research. 2009;**37**(Database issue):D816-D819. DOI: 10.1093/nar/gkn673

[72] Nelson PT, Zhang PJ, Spagnoli GC, Tomaszewski JE, Pasha TL, Frosina D, et al. Cancer/testis (CT) antigens are expressed in fetal ovary. Cancer Immunity. 2007;7:1

[73] Jungbluth AA, Silva WA Jr, Iversen K, Frosina D, Zaidi B, Coplan K, et al. Expression of cancer-testis (CT) antigens in placenta. Cancer Immunity. 2007;7:15

[74] Simpson AJ, Caballero OL, Jungbluth A, Chen YT, Old LJ. Cancer/testis antigens, gametogenesis and cancer. Nature Reviews Cancer. 2005;**5**(8):615-625. DOI: 10.1038/nrc1669

[75] Ross MT, Grafham DV, Coffey AJ, Scherer S, McLay K, Muzny D, et al. The DNA sequence of the human X chromosome. Nature. 2005;**434**(7031):325-337. DOI: 10.1038/nature03440

[76] Chen Y-T, Iseli C, Venditti CA, Old LJ, Simpson AJG, Jongeneel CV. Identification of a new cancer/testis gene family, CT47, among expressed multicopy genes on the human X chromosome. Genes, Chromosomes & Cancer. 2006;**45**(4):392-400. DOI: 10.1002/gcc.20298

[77] Goydos JS, Patel M, Shih W. NY-ESO-1 and CTp11 expression may correlate with stage of progression in melanoma. The Journal of Surgical Research. 2001;**98**(2):76-80. DOI: 10.1006/jsre.2001.6148

[78] Brasseur F, Rimoldi D, Liénard D, Lethé B, Carrel S, Arienti F, et al. Expression of MAGE genes in primary and metastatic cutaneous melanoma. International Journal of Cancer. 1995;**63**(3):375-380. DOI: 10.1002/ijc.2910630313

[79] Velazquez EF, Jungbluth AA, Yancovitz M, Gnjatic S, Adams S, O'Neill D, et al. Expression of the cancer/testis antigen NY-ESO-1 in primary and metastatic malignant melanoma (MM)—Correlation with prognostic factors. Cancer Immunity. 2007;7:11

[80] Svobodová S, Browning J, MacGregor D, Pollara G, Scolyer R, Murali R, et al. Cancer–testis antigen expression in primary cutaneous melanoma has independent prognostic value comparable to that of Breslow thickness, ulceration and mitotic rate *. European Journal of Cancer (Oxford, England: 1990). 2011;**47**:460-469. DOI: 10.1016/j.ejca.2010.09.042

[81] Badal B, Solovyov A, Di Cecilia S, Chan JM, Chang L-W, Iqbal R, et al. Transcriptional dissection of melanoma identifies a high-risk subtype underlying TP53 family genes and epigenome deregulation. JCI Insight [Internet]. 2017;**2**(9):e92102. DOI: 10.1172/jci.insight.92102

[82] Szklarczyk D, Franceschini A, Wyder S, Forslund K, Heller D, Huerta-Cepas J, et al. STRING v10: Protein-protein interaction networks, integrated over the tree of life. Nucleic Acids Research. 2015;**43**(Database issue):D447-D452. DOI: 10.1093/nar/gku1003

[83] Epping MT, Wang L, Edel MJ, Carlée L, Hernandez M, Bernards R. The human tumor antigen PRAME is a dominant repressor of retinoic acid receptor signaling. Cell. 2005;**122**(6):835-847. DOI: 10.1016/j.cell.2005.07.003

[84] Yang B, O'Herrin SM, Wu J, Reagan-Shaw S, Ma Y, Bhat KM, et al. MAGE-A, mMage-b, and MAGE-C

proteins form complexes with KAP1 and suppress p53-dependent apoptosis in MAGE-positive cell lines. Cancer Research. 2007;**67**(20):9954-9962. DOI: 10.1158/0008-5472.can-07-1478

[85] Monte M, Simonatto M, Peche LY, Bublik DR, Gobessi S, Pierotti MA, et al. MAGE-A tumor antigens target p53 transactivation function through histone deacetylase recruitment and confer resistance to chemotherapeutic agents. Proceedings of the National Academy of Sciences of the United States of America. 2006;**103**(30):11160-11165. DOI: 10.1073/pnas.0510834103

[86] Peche LY, Scolz M, Ladelfa MF, Monte M, Schneider C. MageA2 restrains cellular senescence by targeting the function of PMLIV/p53 axis at the PML-NBs. Cell Death and Differentiation. 2012;**19**(6):926-936. DOI: 10.1038/cdd.2011.173

[87] Pearson M, Carbone R, Sebastiani C, Cioce M, Fagioli M, Saito S, et al. PML regulates p53 acetylation and premature senescence induced by oncogenic Ras. Nature. 2000;**406**(6792):207-210. DOI: 10.1038/35018127

[88] Baylin SB, Herman JG. DNA hypermethylation in tumorigenesis: Epigenetics joins genetics. Trends in Genetics: TIG. 2000;**16**(4):168-174. DOI: 10.1016/s0168-9525(99)01971-x

[89] Kimmins S, Sassone-Corsi P. Chromatin remodelling and epigenetic features of germ cells. Nature. 2005;**434**(7033):583-589. DOI: 10.1038/nature03368

[90] De Smet C, Lurquin C, Lethé B, Martelange V, Boon T. DNA methylation is the primary silencing mechanism for a set of germ line- and tumor-specific genes with a CpG-rich promoter. Molecular and Cellular Biology. 1999;**19**(11):7327-7335. DOI: 10.1128/mcb.19.11.7327

[91] Coral S, Sigalotti L, Altomonte M, Engelsberg A, Colizzi F, Cattarossi I, et al. 5-Aza-2′-deoxycytidine-induced expression of functional cancer testis antigens in human renal cell carcinoma: Immunotherapeutic implications. Clinical Cancer Research: An Official Journal of the American Association for Cancer Research. 2002;**8**(8):2690-2695

[92] Old LJ. Cancer/testis (CT) antigens—A new link between gametogenesis and cancer. Cancer Immunity. 2001;**1**:1

[93] Kalejs M, Erenpreisa J. Cancer/testis antigens and gametogenesis: A review and "brain-storming" session. Cancer Cell International. 2005;**5**(1):4. DOI: 10.1186/1475-2867-5-4

[94] Lee AK, Potts PR. A comprehensive guide to the MAGE family of ubiquitin ligases. Journal of Molecular Biology. 2017;**429**(8):1114-1142. DOI: 10.1016/j.jmb.2017.03.005

[95] Lipkowitz S, Weissman AM. RINGs of good and evil: RING finger ubiquitin ligases at the crossroads of tumour suppression and oncogenesis. Nature Reviews Cancer. 2011;**11**(9):629-643. DOI: 10.1038/nrc3120

[96] Kouprina N, Mullokandov M, Rogozin IB, Collins NK, Solomon G, Otstot J, et al. The SPANX gene family of cancer/testis-specific antigens: Rapid evolution and amplification in African great apes and hominids. Proceedings of the National Academy of Sciences of the United States of America. 2004;**101**(9):3077-3082. DOI: 10.1073/pnas.0308532100

[97] Rajagopalan K, Mooney SM, Parekh N, Getzenberg RH, Kulkarni P. A majority of the cancer/testis antigens are intrinsically disordered proteins. Journal of Cellular Biochemistry.

2011;**112**(11):3256-3267. DOI: 10.1002/jcb.23252

[98] Dunker AK, Cortese MS, Romero P, Iakoucheva LM, Uversky VN. Flexible nets. The roles of intrinsic disorder in protein interaction networks. The FEBS Journal. 2005;**272**(20):5129-5148. DOI: 10.1111/j.1742-4658.2005.04948.x

[99] Radivojac P, Iakoucheva LM, Oldfield CJ, Obradovic Z, Uversky VN, Dunker AK. Intrinsic disorder and functional proteomics. Biophysical Journal. 2007;**92**(5):1439-1456. DOI: 10.1529/biophysj.106.094045

[100] Darling AL, Uversky VN. Intrinsic disorder and posttranslational modifications: The darker side of the biological dark matter. Frontiers in Genetics. 2018;**9**:158. DOI: 10.3389/fgene.2018.00158

[101] Giuliani A, Di Paola L. The two faces of protein flexibility: A topological approach. Current Chemical Biology. 2018;**12**:14. DOI: 10.2174/2212796811666170717113552

[102] Tanner MM, Grenman S, Koul A, Johannsson O, Meltzer P, Pejovic T, et al. Frequent amplification of chromosomal region 20q12-q13 in ovarian cancer. Clinical Cancer Research: An Official Journal of the American Association for Cancer Research. 2000;**6**(5):1833-1839

[103] Hidaka S, Yasutake T, Takeshita H, Kondo M, Tsuji T, Nanashima A, et al. Differences in 20q13.2 copy number between colorectal cancers with and without liver metastasis. Clinical Cancer Research: An Official Journal of the American Association for Cancer Research. 2000;**6**(7):2712-2717

[104] Loukinov DI, Pugacheva E, Vatolin S, Pack SD, Moon H, Chernukhin I, et al. BORIS, a novel male germ-line-specific protein associated with epigenetic reprogramming events, shares the same 11-zinc-finger domain with CTCF, the insulator protein involved in reading imprinting marks in the soma. Proceedings of the National Academy of Sciences of the United States of America. 2002;**99**(10):6806-6811. DOI: 10.1073/pnas.092123699

[105] Kholmanskikh O, Loriot A, Brasseur F, De Plaen E, De Smet C. Expression of BORIS in melanoma: Lack of association with MAGE-A1 activation. International Journal of Cancer. 2008;**122**(4):777-784. DOI: 10.1002/ijc.23140

[106] Klenova EM, Morse HC 3rd, Ohlsson R, Lobanenkov VV. The novel BORIS + CTCF gene family is uniquely involved in the epigenetics of normal biology and cancer. Seminars in Cancer Biology. 2002;**12**(5):399-414. DOI: 10.1016/s1044-579x(02)00060-3

[107] Janssen SM, Moscona R, Elchebly M, Papadakis AI, Redpath M, Wang H, et al. BORIS/CTCFL promotes a switch from a proliferative towards an invasive phenotype in melanoma cells. Cell Death Discovery. 2020;**6**:1. DOI: 10.1038/s41420-019-0235-x

[108] Phillips JE, Corces VG. CTCF: Master weaver of the genome. Cell. 2009;**137**(7):1194-1211. DOI: 10.1016/j.cell.2009.06.001

[109] Marshall AD, Bailey CG, Rasko JE. CTCF and BORIS in genome regulation and cancer. Current Opinion in Genetics & Development. 2014;**24**:8-15. DOI: 10.1016/j.gde.2013.10.011

[110] Smith IM, Glazer CA, Mithani SK, Ochs MF, Sun W, Bhan S, et al. Coordinated activation of candidate proto-oncogenes and cancer testes antigens via promoter demethylation in head and neck cancer and lung cancer. PLoS One. 2009;**4**(3):e4961. DOI: 10.1371/journal.pone.0004961

[111] Renaud S, Loukinov D, Alberti L, Vostrov A, Kwon YW,

Bosman FT, et al. BORIS/CTCFL-mediated transcriptional regulation of the hTERT telomerase gene in testicular and ovarian tumor cells. Nucleic Acids Research. 2011;**39**(3):862-873. DOI: 10.1093/nar/gkq827

[112] Liu Q, Chen K, Liu Z, Huang Y, Zhao R, Wei L, et al. BORIS up-regulates OCT4 via histone methylation to promote cancer stem cell-like properties in human liver cancer cells. Cancer Letters. 2017;**403**:165-174. DOI: 10.1016/j.canlet.2017.06.017

[113] Zampieri M, Ciccarone F, Palermo R, Cialfi S, Passananti C, Chiaretti S, et al. The epigenetic factor BORIS/CTCFL regulates the NOTCH3 gene expression in cancer cells. Biochimica et Biophysica Acta. 2014;**1839**(9):813-825. DOI: 10.1016/j.bbagrm.2014.06.017

[114] Nguyen P, Bar-Sela G, Sun L, Bisht KS, Cui H, Kohn E, et al. BAT3 and SET1A form a complex with CTCFL/BORIS to modulate H3K4 histone dimethylation and gene expression. Molecular and Cellular Biology. 2008;**28**(21):6720-6729. DOI: 10.1128/mcb.00568-08

[115] Sun L, Huang L, Nguyen P, Bisht KS, Bar-Sela G, Ho AS, et al. DNA methyltransferase 1 and 3B activate BAG-1 expression via recruitment of CTCFL/BORIS and modulation of promoter histone methylation. Cancer Research. 2008;**68**(8):2726-2735. DOI: 10.1158/0008-5472.can-07-6654

[116] Kosaka-Suzuki N, Suzuki T, Pugacheva EM, Vostrov AA, Morse HC 3rd, Loukinov D, et al. Transcription factor BORIS (Brother of the Regulator of Imprinted Sites) directly induces expression of a cancer-testis antigen, TSP50, through regulated binding of BORIS to the promoter. The Journal of Biological Chemistry. 2011;**286**(31):27378-27388. DOI: 10.1074/jbc.M111.243576

[117] Vatolin S, Abdullaev Z, Pack SD, Flanagan PT, Custer M, Loukinov DI, et al. Conditional expression of the CTCF-paralogous transcriptional factor BORIS in normal cells results in demethylation and derepression of MAGE-A1 and reactivation of other cancer-testis genes. Cancer Research. 2005;**65**(17):7751-7762. DOI: 10.1158/0008-5472.can-05-0858

[118] Hillman J, Pugacheva E, Barger C, Sribenja S, Rosario S, Albahrani M, et al. BORIS expression in ovarian cancer precursor cells alters the CTCF cistrome and enhances invasiveness through GALNT14. Molecular Cancer Research. 2019;**17**(10):2051-2062. DOI: 10.1158/1541-7786.MCR-19-0310

[119] Alberti L, Losi L, Leyvraz S, Benhattar J. Different effects of BORIS/CTCFL on stemness gene expression, sphere formation and cell survival in epithelial cancer stem cells. PLoS One. 2015;**10**(7):e0132977. DOI: 10.1371/journal.pone.0132977

[120] Alberti L, Renaud S, Losi L, Leyvraz S, Benhattar J. High expression of hTERT and stemness genes in BORIS/CTCFL positive cells isolated from embryonic cancer cells. PLoS One. 2014;**9**(10):e109921. DOI: 10.1371/journal.pone.0109921

[121] Link PA, Zhang W, Odunsi K, Karpf AR. BORIS/CTCFL mRNA isoform expression and epigenetic regulation in epithelial ovarian cancer. Cancer Immunity. 2013;**13**:6

[122] Murakami S, Ninomiya W, Sakamoto E, Shibata T, Akiyama H, Tashiro F. SRY and OCT4 are required for the acquisition of cancer stem cell-like properties and are potential differentiation therapy targets. Stem Cells (Dayton, Ohio). 2015;**33**(9):2652-2663. DOI: 10.1002/stem.2059

[123] Kumar SM, Liu S, Lu H, Zhang H, Zhang PJ, Gimotty PA, et al. Acquired

cancer stem cell phenotypes through Oct4-mediated dedifferentiation. Oncogene. 2012;**31**(47):4898-4911. DOI: 10.1038/onc.2011.656

[124] Wang YJ, Herlyn M. The emerging roles of Oct4 in tumor-initiating cells. American Journal of Physiology-Cell Physiology. 2015;**309**(11):C709-C718. DOI: 10.1152/ajpcell.00212.2015

[125] Zhao W, Li Y, Zhang X. Stemness-related markers in cancer. Cancer Translational Medicine. 2017;**3**(3):87-95. DOI: 10.4103/ctm.ctm_69_16

[126] Colaprico A, Silva TC, Olsen C, Garofano L, Cava C, Garolini D, et al. TCGAbiolinks: An R/Bioconductor package for integrative analysis of TCGA data. Nucleic Acids Research. 2016;**44**(8):e71. DOI: 10.1093/nar/gkv1507

[127] Robinson MD, McCarthy DJ, Smyth GK. edgeR: A Bioconductor package for differential expression analysis of digital gene expression data. Bioinformatics (Oxford, England). 2010;**26**(1):139-140. DOI: 10.1093/bioinformatics/btp616

[128] Waskom MB, Olga O, Kane HD, Lukauskas P, Gemperline S, et al. Seaborn. v0.8. 1st ed. Internet. Meyrin, Switzerland: Zenodo; 2017

[129] Boregowda RK, Medina DJ, Markert E, Bryan MA, Chen W, Chen S, et al. The transcription factor RUNX2 regulates receptor tyrosine kinase expression in melanoma. Oncotarget. 2016;**7**(20):29689-29707. DOI: 10.18632/oncotarget.8822

[130] Sinnberg T, Levesque MP, Krochmann J, Cheng PF, Ikenberg K, Meraz-Torres F, et al. Wnt-signaling enhances neural crest migration of melanoma cells and induces an invasive phenotype. Molecular Cancer. 2018;**17**(1):59. DOI: 10.1186/s12943-018-0773-5

[131] McFarlane RJ, Wakeman JA. Meiosis-like functions in oncogenesis: A new view of cancer. Cancer Research. 2017;**77**(21):5712-5716. DOI: 10.1158/0008-5472.can-17-1535

[132] Keeney S, Giroux CN, Kleckner N. Meiosis-specific DNA double-strand breaks are catalyzed by Spo11, a member of a widely conserved protein family. Cell. 1997;**88**(3):375-384. DOI: 10.1016/s0092-8674(00)81876-0

[133] Baudat F, Manova K, Yuen JP, Jasin M, Keeney S. Chromosome synapsis defects and sexually dimorphic meiotic progression in mice lacking Spo11. Molecular Cell. 2000;**6**(5):989-998. DOI: 10.1016/s1097-2765(00)00098-8

[134] Romanienko PJ, Camerini-Otero RD. The mouse Spo11 gene is required for meiotic chromosome synapsis. Molecular Cell. 2000;**6**(5):975-987. DOI: 10.1016/s1097-2765(00)00097-6

[135] Koslowski M, Türeci O, Bell C, Krause P, Lehr HA, Brunner J, et al. Multiple splice variants of lactate dehydrogenase C selectively expressed in human cancer. Cancer Research. 2002;**62**(22):6750-6755

[136] Atanackovic D, Luetkens T, Kloth B, Fuchs G, Cao Y, Hildebrandt Y, et al. Cancer-testis antigen expression and its epigenetic modulation in acute myeloid leukemia. American Journal of Hematology. 2011;**86**(11):918-922. DOI: 10.1002/ajh.22141

[137] Litvinov IV, Cordeiro B, Huang Y, Zargham H, Pehr K, Doré MA, et al. Ectopic expression of cancer-testis antigens in cutaneous T-cell lymphoma patients. Clinical Cancer Research: An Official Journal of the American Association for Cancer Research. 2014;**20**(14):3799-3808. DOI: 10.1158/1078-0432.ccr-14-0307

[138] Eldai H, Periyasamy S, Al Qarni S, Al Rodayyan M, Muhammed Mustafa S,

Deeb A, et al. Novel genes associated with colorectal cancer are revealed by high resolution cytogenetic analysis in a patient specific manner. PLoS One. 2013;**8**(10):e76251. DOI: 10.1371/journal.pone.0076251

[139] Tsang M, Gantchev J, Netchiporouk E, Moreau L, Ghazawi FM, Glassman S, et al. A study of meiomitosis and novel pathways of genomic instability in cutaneous T-cell lymphomas (CTCL). Oncotarget. 2018;**9**(102):37647-37661. DOI: 10.18632/oncotarget.26479

[140] Kim S, Peterson SE, Jasin M, Keeney S. Mechanisms of germ line genome instability. Seminars in Cell & Developmental Biology. 2016;**54**:177-187. DOI: 10.1016/j.semcdb.2016.02.019

[141] Nagirnaja L, Aston KI, Conrad DF. Genetic intersection of male infertility and cancer. Fertility and Sterility. 2018;**109**(1):20-26. DOI: 10.1016/j.fertnstert.2017.10.028

[142] Dernburg AF, McDonald K, Moulder G, Barstead R, Dresser M, Villeneuve AM. Meiotic recombination in *C. elegans* initiates by a conserved mechanism and is dispensable for homologous chromosome synapsis. Cell. 1998;**94**(3):387-398. DOI: 10.1016/s0092-8674(00)81481-6

[143] Keeney S. Spo11 and the formation of DNA double-strand breaks in meiosis. Genome Dynamics and Stability. 2008;**2**:81-123. DOI: 10.1007/7050_2007_026

[144] Klein U, Esposito G, Baudat F, Keeney S, Jasin M. Mice deficient for the type II topoisomerase-like DNA transesterase Spo11 show normal immunoglobulin somatic hypermutation and class switching. European Journal of Immunology. 2002;**32**(2):316-321. DOI: 10.1002/1521-4141(200202)32:2<316::aid-immu316>3.0.co;2-p

[145] Prieler S, Penkner A, Borde V, Klein F. The control of Spo11's interaction with meiotic recombination hotspots. Genes & Development. 2005;**19**(2):255-269. DOI: 10.1101/gad.321105

[146] Huna A, Salmina K, Erenpreisa J, Vazquez-Martin A, Krigerts J, Inashkina I, et al. Role of stress-activated OCT4A in the cell fate decisions of embryonal carcinoma cells treated with etoposide. Cell Cycle (Georgetown, Texas). 2015;**14**(18):2969-2984. DOI: 10.1080/15384101.2015.1056948

[147] Tock AJ, Henderson IR. Hotspots for initiation of meiotic recombination. Frontiers in Genetics. 2018;**9**:521. DOI: 10.3389/fgene.2018.00521

[148] Neale MJ, Pan J, Keeney S. Endonucleolytic processing of covalent protein-linked DNA double-strand breaks. Nature. 2005;**436**(7053):1053-1057. DOI: 10.1038/nature03872

[149] Bomblies K, Higgins JD, Yant L. Meiosis evolves: Adaptation to external and internal environments. New Phytologist. 2015;**208**(2):306-323. DOI: 10.1111/nph.13499

[150] Yant L, Bomblies K. Genome management and mismanagement--cell-level opportunities and challenges of whole-genome duplication. Genes & Development. 2015;**29**(23):2405-2419. DOI: 10.1101/gad.271072.115

[151] Feichtinger J, Aldeailej I, Anderson R, Almutairi M, Almatrafi A, Alsiwiehri N, et al. Meta-analysis of clinical data using human meiotic genes identifies a novel cohort of highly restricted cancer-specific marker genes. Oncotarget. 2012;**3**(8):843-853. DOI: 10.18632/oncotarget.580

[152] Loriot A, Boon T, De Smet C. Five new human cancer-germline genes

identified among 12 genes expressed in spermatogonia. International Journal of Cancer. 2003;**105**(3):371-376. DOI: 10.1002/ijc.11104

[153] Liu JG, Yuan L, Brundell E, Björkroth B, Daneholt B, Höög C. Localization of the N-terminus of SCP1 to the central element of the synaptonemal complex and evidence for direct interactions between the N-termini of SCP1 molecules organized head-to-head. Experimental Cell Research. 1996;**226**(1):11-19. DOI: 10.1006/excr.1996.0197

[154] Schmekel K, Meuwissen RL, Dietrich AJ, Vink AC, van Marle J, van Veen H, et al. Organization of SCP1 protein molecules within synaptonemal complexes of the rat. Experimental Cell Research. 1996;**226**(1):20-30. DOI: 10.1006/excr.1996.0198

[155] Ollinger R, Alsheimer M, Benavente R. Mammalian protein SCP1 forms synaptonemal complex-like structures in the absence of meiotic chromosomes. Molecular Biology of the Cell. 2005;**16**(1):212-217. DOI: 10.1091/mbc.e04-09-0771

[156] Costa Y, Speed R, Ollinger R, Alsheimer M, Semple CA, Gautier P, et al. Two novel proteins recruited by synaptonemal complex protein 1 (SYCP1) are at the Centre of meiosis. Journal of Cell Science 2005; 118 (Pt 12):2755-2762. doi:10.1242/jcs.02402

[157] Türeci O, Sahin U, Zwick C, Koslowski M, Seitz G, Pfreundschuh M. Identification of a meiosis-specific protein as a member of the class of cancer/testis antigens. Proceedings of the National Academy of Sciences of the United States of America. 1998;**95**(9):5211-5216. DOI: 10.1073/pnas.95.9.5211

[158] Mobasheri MB, Jahanzad I, Mohagheghi MA, Aarabi M, Farzan S, Modarressi MH. Expression of two testis-specific genes, TSGA10 and SYCP3, in different cancers regarding to their pathological features. Cancer Detection and Prevention. 2007;**31**(4):296-302. DOI: 10.1016/j.cdp.2007.05.002

[159] Cho H, Noh KH, Chung JY, Takikita M, Chung EJ, Kim BW, et al. Synaptonemal complex protein 3 is a prognostic marker in cervical cancer. PLoS One. 2014;**9**(6):e98712. DOI: 10.1371/journal.pone.0098712

[160] Chung JY, Kitano H, Takikita M, Cho H, Noh KH, Kim TW, et al. Synaptonemal complex protein 3 as a novel prognostic marker in early stage non-small cell lung cancer. Human Pathology. 2013;**44**(4):472-479. DOI: 10.1016/j.humpath.2012.06.018

[161] Daniel K, Lange J, Hached K, Fu J, Anastassiadis K, Roig I, et al. Meiotic homologue alignment and its quality surveillance are controlled by mouse HORMAD1. Nature Cell Biology. 2011;**13**(5):599-610. DOI: 10.1038/ncb2213

[162] Yao J, Caballero OL, Yung WK, Weinstein JN, Riggins GJ, Strausberg RL, et al. Tumor subtype-specific cancer-testis antigens as potential biomarkers and immunotherapeutic targets for cancers. Cancer Immunology Research. 2014;**2**(4):371-379. DOI: 10.1158/2326-6066.cir-13-0088

[163] Nichols BA, Oswald NW, McMillan EA, McGlynn K, Yan J, Kim MS, et al. HORMAD1 is a negative prognostic indicator in lung adenocarcinoma and specifies resistance to oxidative and genotoxic stress. Cancer Research. 2018;**78**(21):6196-6208. DOI: 10.1158/0008-5472.can-18-1377

[164] Wang X, Tan Y, Cao X, Kim JA, Chen T, Hu Y, et al. Epigenetic activation of HORMAD1 in basal-like breast cancer: Role in rucaparib sensitivity.

Oncotarget. 2018;**9**(53):30115-30127. DOI: 10.18632/oncotarget.25728

[165] Ishiguro KI. The cohesin complex in mammalian meiosis. Genes to Cells: Devoted to Molecular & Cellular Mechanisms. 2019;**24**(1):6-30. DOI: 10.1111/gtc.12652

[166] Rosa AM, Dabas N, Byrnes DM, Eller MS, Grichnik JM. Germ cell proteins in melanoma: Prognosis, diagnosis, treatment, and theories on expression. Journal of Skin Cancer. 2012;**2012**:621968. DOI: 10.1155/2012/621968

[167] Gantchev J, Martínez Villarreal A, Xie P, Lefrançois P, Gunn S, Netchiporouk E, et al. The ectopic expression of meiosis regulatory genes in cutaneous T-cell lymphomas (CTCL). Frontiers in Oncology. 2019;**9**:429. DOI: 10.3389/fonc.2019.00429

[168] Erenpreisa J, Cragg MS, Salmina K, Hausmann M, Scherthan H. The role of meiotic cohesin REC8 in chromosome segregation in gamma irradiation-induced endopolyploid tumour cells. Experimental Cell Research. 2009;**315**(15):2593-2603. DOI: 10.1016/j.yexcr.2009.05.011

[169] Folco HD, Chalamcharla VR, Sugiyama T, Thillainadesan G, Zofall M, Balachandran V, et al. Untimely expression of gametogenic genes in vegetative cells causes uniparental disomy. Nature. 2017;**543**(7643):126-130. DOI: 10.1038/nature21372

[170] Wolf PG, Cuba Ramos A, Kenzel J, Neumann B, Stemmann O. Studying meiotic cohesin in somatic cells reveals that Rec8-containing cohesin requires Stag3 to function and is regulated by Wapl and sororin. Journal of Cell Science. 2018;**131**(11):jcs212100. DOI: 10.1242/jcs.212100

[171] Shen CH, Kim SH, Trousil S, Frederick DT, Piris A, Yuan P, et al. Loss of cohesin complex components STAG2 or STAG3 confers resistance to BRAF inhibition in melanoma. Nature Medicine. 2016;**22**(9):1056-1061. DOI: 10.1038/nm.4155

[172] Brar GA, Amon A. Emerging roles for centromeres in meiosis I chromosome segregation. Nature Reviews Genetics. 2008;**9**(12):899-910. DOI: 10.1038/nrg2454

[173] Eijpe M, Offenberg H, Jessberger R, Revenkova E, Heyting C. Meiotic cohesin REC8 marks the axial elements of rat synaptonemal complexes before cohesins SMC1beta and SMC3. The Journal of Cell Biology. 2003;**160**(5):657-670. DOI: 10.1083/jcb.200212080

[174] Kitajima TS, Sakuno T, Ishiguro K, Iemura S, Natsume T, Kawashima SA, et al. Shugoshin collaborates with protein phosphatase 2A to protect cohesin. Nature. 2006;**441**(7089):46-52. DOI: 10.1038/nature04663

[175] Herrán Y, Gutiérrez-Caballero C, Sanchez-Martin M, Hernández T, Viera A, Barbero J, et al. The cohesin subunit RAD21L functions in meiotic synapsis and exhibits sexual dimorphism in fertility. The EMBO Journal. 2011;**30**:3091-3105. DOI: 10.1038/emboj.2011.222

[176] De Vitis M, Berardinelli F, Sgura A. Telomere length maintenance in cancer: At the crossroad between telomerase and alternative lengthening of telomeres (ALT). International Journal of Molecular Sciences. 2018;**19**(2):606. DOI: 10.3390/ijms19020606

[177] Salmina K, Bojko A, Inashkina I, Staniak K, Dudkowska M, Podlesniy P, et al. "mitotic slippage" and extranuclear DNA in cancer chemoresistance: A focus on telomeres. International Journal of Molecular Sciences. 2020;**21**(8):2779. DOI: 10.3390/ijms21082779

[178] Cho NW, Dilley RL, Lampson MA, Greenberg RA. Interchromosomal homology searches drive directional ALT telomere movement and synapsis. Cell. 2014;**159**(1):108-121. DOI: 10.1016/j.cell.2014.08.030

[179] Rong M, Miyauchi S, Lee J. Ectopic expression of meiotic cohesin RAD21L promotes adjacency of homologous chromosomes in somatic cells. The Journal of Reproduction and Development. 2017;**63**(3):227-234. DOI: 10.1262/jrd.2016-171

[180] Dilley RL, Verma P, Cho NW, Winters HD, Wondisford AR, Greenberg RA. Break-induced telomere synthesis underlies alternative telomere maintenance. Nature. 2016;**539**(7627):54-58. DOI: 10.1038/nature20099

[181] Dobzhansky T. Nothing in biology makes sense except in the light of evolution. The American Biology Teacher. 1973;**35**(3):125-129. DOI: 10.2307/4444260

[182] Weinberg RA. Coming full circle-from endless complexity to simplicity and back again. Cell. 2014;**157**(1):267-271. DOI: 10.1016/j.cell.2014.03.004

[183] Lee S, Schmitt CA. The dynamic nature of senescence in cancer. Nature Cell Biology. 2019;**21**(1):94-101. DOI: 10.1038/s41556-018-0249-2

[184] Grichnik JM. Genomic instability and tumor stem cells. The Journal of Investigative Dermatology. 2006;**126**(6):1214-1216. DOI: 10.1038/sj.jid.5700240

[185] Grichnik JM. Melanoma, nevogenesis, and stem cell biology. The Journal of Investigative Dermatology. 2008;**128**(10):2365-2380. DOI: 10.1038/jid.2008.166

[186] Sheltzer JM, Amon A. The aneuploidy paradox: Costs and benefits of an incorrect karyotype. Trends in Genetics: TIG. 2011;**27**(11):446-453. DOI: 10.1016/j.tig.2011.07.003

[187] Muller HJ. The relation of recombination to mutational advance. Mutation Research. 1964;**106**:2-9. DOI: 10.1016/0027-5107(64)90047-8

[188] Neher RA, Shraiman BI. Fluctuations of fitness distributions and the rate of Muller's ratchet. Genetics. 2012;**191**(4):1283-1293. DOI: 10.1534/genetics.112.141325

[189] Amend SR, Torga G, Lin KC, Kostecka LG, de Marzo A, Austin RH, et al. Polyploid giant cancer cells: Unrecognized actuators of tumorigenesis, metastasis, and resistance. The Prostate. 2019;**79**(13):1489-1497. DOI: 10.1002/pros.23877

[190] Coward J, Harding A. Size does matter: Why polyploid tumor cells are critical drug targets in the war on cancer. Frontiers in Oncology. 2014;**4**:123. DOI: 10.3389/fonc.2014.00123

[191] Mirzayans R, Andrais B, Murray D. Roles of polyploid/multinucleated giant cancer cells in metastasis and disease relapse following anticancer treatment. Cancers. 2018;**10**(4):118. DOI: 10.3390/cancers10040118

[192] Chen J, Niu N, Zhang J, Qi L, Shen W, Donkena KV, et al. Polyploid giant cancer cells (PGCCs): The evil roots of cancer. Current Cancer Drug Targets. 2019;**19**(5):360-367. DOI: 10.2174/1568009618666180703154233

[193] Erenpreisa J, Cragg M. Cancer: A matter of life cycle? Cell Biology International. 2007;**31**:1507-1510. DOI: 10.1016/j.cellbi.2007.08.013

[194] Sundaram M, Guernsey DL, Rajaraman MM, Rajaraman R. Neosis: A novel type of cell division in cancer. Cancer Biology & Therapy. 2004;**3**(2):207-218. DOI: 10.4161/cbt.3.2.663

[195] Rajaraman R, Guernsey D, Rajaraman M, Rajaraman S. Neosis—A parasexual somatic reduction division in cancer. International Journal of Human Genetics. 2007;7:29-48. DOI: 10.1080/09723757.2007.11885983

[196] Salmina K, Jankevics E, Huna A, Perminov D, Radovica I, Klymenko T, et al. Up-regulation of the embryonic self-renewal network through reversible polyploidy in irradiated p53-mutant tumour cells. Experimental Cell Research. 2010;**316**(13):2099-2112. DOI: 10.1016/j.yexcr.2010.04.030

[197] Lagadec C, Vlashi E, Della Donna L, Dekmezian C, Pajonk F. Radiation-induced reprogramming of breast cancer cells. Stem Cells (Dayton, Ohio). 2012;**30**(5):833-844. DOI: 10.1002/stem.1058

[198] Mosieniak G, Sikora E. Polyploidy: The link between senescence and cancer. Current Pharmaceutical Design. 2010;**16**(6):734-740. DOI: 10.2174/138161210790883714

[199] Weihua Z, Lin Q, Ramoth AJ, Fan D, Fidler IJ. Formation of solid tumors by a single multinucleated cancer cell. Cancer. 2011;**117**(17):4092-4099. DOI: 10.1002/cncr.26021

[200] Mirzayans R, Andrais B, Murray D. Viability assessment following anticancer treatment requires single-cell visualization. Cancers. 2018;**10**(8):255. DOI: 10.3390/cancers10080255

[201] Erenpreisa J, Cragg M, Fringes B, Sharakhov I. Release of mitotic descendents by giant cells from Burkitt's lymphoma cell line. Cell Biology International. 2000;**24**:635-648. DOI: 10.1006/cbir.2000.0558

[202] Erenpreisa J, Kalejs M, Ianzini F, Kosmacek EA, Mackey MA, Emzinsh D, et al. Segregation of genomes in polyploid tumour cells following mitotic catastrophe. Cell Biology International. 2005;**29**(12):1005-1011. DOI: 10.1016/j.cellbi.2005.10.008

[203] Comai L. The advantages and disadvantages of being polyploid. Nature Reviews Genetics. 2005;**6**(11):836-846. DOI: 10.1038/nrg1711

[204] Markov AV, Kaznacheev IS. Evolutionary consequences of polyploidy in prokaryotes and the origin of mitosis and meiosis. Biology Direct. 2016;**11**:28. DOI: 10.1186/s13062-016-0131-8

[205] Bernstein H, Byerly HC, Hopf FA, Michod R. DNA Repair and complementation: The major factors in the origin and maintenance of sex. In: Halvorson HO, Monroy A, editors. The Origin and Evolution of Sex. New York: Alan R.Liss Inc.; 1985. pp. 29-45

[206] Kondrashov AS. The asexual ploidy cycle and the origin of sex. Nature. 1994;**370**(6486):213-216. DOI: 10.1038/370213a0

[207] Erenpreisa J, Kalejs M, Cragg MS. Mitotic catastrophe and endomitosis in tumour cells: An evolutionary key to a molecular solution. Cell Biology International. 2005;**29**(12):1012-1018. DOI: 10.1016/j.cellbi.2005.10.005

[208] Cleveland LR. The origin and evolution of meiosis. Science (New York, N.Y.). 1947;**105**(2724):287-289. DOI: 10.1126/science.105.2724.287

[209] Solari AJ. Primitive forms of meiosis: The possible evolution of meiosis. Biocell. 2002;**26**(1):1-13

[210] Loidl J. Conservation and variability of meiosis across the eukaryotes. Annual Review of Genetics. 2016;**50**:293-316. DOI: 10.1146/annurev-genet-120215-035100

[211] Bogdanov Y. Variation and evolution of meiosis. Russian Journal of Genetics. 2003;**39**:363-381

[212] Old LJ. Cancer is a somatic cell pregnancy. Cancer Immunity. 2007;**7**:19

[213] Erenpreisa J, Salmina K, Huna A, Jackson TR, Vazquez-Martin A, Cragg MS. The "virgin birth", polyploidy, and the origin of cancer. Oncoscience. 2015;**2**(1):3-14. DOI: 10.18632/oncoscience.108

[214] Liu J. The "life code": A theory that unifies the human life cycle and the origin of human tumors. Seminars in Cancer Biology. 2020;**60**:380-397. DOI: 10.1016/j.semcancer.2019.09.005

[215] Vainshelbaum NM, Zayakin P, Kleina R, Giuliani A, Erenpreisa J. Meta-analysis of cancer triploidy: Rearrangements of genome complements in male human tumors are characterized by XXY karyotypes. Genes. 2019;**10**(8):613. DOI: 10.3390/genes10080613

[216] Salmina K, Gerashchenko B, Hausmann VN, Zayakin E, et al. When three isn't a crowd: A digyny concept for treatment-resistant, near-triploid human cancers. Genes. 2019;**10**:551. DOI: 10.3390/genes10070551

[217] Huskins CL, Cheng KC. Segregation and reduction in somatic tissues: IV. Reductional groupings induced in *Allium cepa* by low temperature. Journal of Heredity. 1950;**41**(1):13-18. DOI: 10.1093/oxfordjournals.jhered.a106043

[218] Walen K. Neoplastic-like cell changes of normal fibroblast cells associated with evolutionary conserved maternal and paternal genomic autonomous behavior (Gonomery). Journal of Cancer Therapy. 2014;**05**:860-877. DOI: 10.4236/jct.2014.59094

[219] Trigos AS, Pearson RB, Papenfuss AT, Goode DL. Altered interactions between unicellular and multicellular genes drive hallmarks of transformation in a diverse range of solid tumors. Proceedings of the National Academy of Sciences of the United States of America. 2017;**114**(24):6406-6411. DOI: 10.1073/pnas.1617743114

[220] Erenpreisa J, Giuliani A, Vinogradov A, Anatskaya O, Vazquez-Martin A, Salmina K, et al. Stress-induced polyploidy shifts somatic cells towards a pro-tumourogenic unicellular gene transcription network hypothesis: Polyploidy enables access to transcriptional networks of unicellular organisms, which in the absence of tumour suppressors provides immortality and resistance from treatment for cancer cells. Cancer Hypotheses. 2018;**1**:1-20

[221] Heckmann S, Jankowska M, Schubert V, Kumke K, Ma W, Houben A. Alternative meiotic chromatid segregation in the holocentric plant Luzula elegans. Nature Communications. 2014;**5**(1):4979. DOI: 10.1038/ncomms5979

[222] Ottolini CS, Newnham L, Capalbo A, Natesan SA, Joshi HA, Cimadomo D, et al. Genome wide maps of recombination and chromosome segregation in human oocytes and embryos show selection for maternal recombination rates. Nature Genetics. 2015;**47**(7):727-735. DOI: 10.1038/ng.3306

[223] Domazet-Lošo T, Klimovich A, Anokhin B, Anton-Erxleben F, Hamm MJ, Lange C, et al. Naturally occurring tumours in the basal metazoan Hydra. Nature Communications [Internet]. 2014;**5**:4222. DOI: 10.1038/ncomms5222

[224] Erenpreisa J, Giuliani A. Resolution of complex issues in genome regulation and cancer requires non-linear and network-based thermodynamics.

International Journal of Molecular Sciences. 2019;**21**(1):240. DOI: 10.3390/ijms21010240

[225] Huang S, Ernberg I, Kauffman S. Cancer attractors: A systems view of tumors from a gene network dynamics and developmental perspective. Seminars in Cell & Developmental Biology. 2009;**20**(7):869-876. DOI: 10.1016/j.semcdb.2009.07.003

[226] Huang S, Eichler G, Bar-Yam Y, Ingber DE. Cell fates as high-dimensional attractor states of a complex gene regulatory network. Physical Review Letters. 2005;**94**(12): 128701. DOI: 10.1103/PhysRevLett.94.128701

[227] López S, Lim EL, Horswell S. et al. Polyploidy in cancer produces the buffering effect decreasing the homozygous loss. Interplay between whole-genome doubling and the accumulation of deleterious alterations in cancer evolution. Nature Genetics. 2020;**52**:283-293. Available from: http://sci-hub.tw/10.1038/s41588-020-0584-7

[228] Hu T, Kumar Y, Shazia I, Duan S-J, Li Y, Chen L, et al. Forward and reverse mutations in stages of cancer development. Human Genomics. 2018;**12**(1):40. DOI: 10.1186/s40246-018-0170-6

[229] Maciver SK. Asexual amoebae escape Muller's ratchet through polyploidy. Trends in Parasitology. 2016;**32**(11):855-862. DOI: 10.1016/j.pt.2016.08.006

[230] Chen JM, Férec C, Cooper DN. Gene conversion in human genetic disease. Genes. 2010;**1**(3):550-563. DOI: 10.3390/genes1030550

Chapter 7

Role of RUNX2 in Melanoma: A New Player in Tumor Progression and Resistance to Therapy

Rachael Pulica, Karine Cohen Solal and Ahmed Lasfar

Abstract

RUNX2, a transcription factor, initially known for its indispensable role in skeletal development. RUNX2 is essential for osteoblast differentiation and the maintain of the osteocyte balance. RUNX2 acts directly on osteoblasts via Fgf pathway or on mesenchymal progenitors through Hedgehog, Wnt, Pthlh and DLX5. Currently, many reports point its critical role in the progression and metastasis of several cancer types. RUNX2 is involved in EMT process, invasion and metastasis through the modulation of important oncogenic pathways, including Wnt, FAK/PTK and AKT. In melanoma, RUNX2 is a key player in mediating intrinsic RTK-associated pro-oncogenic properties. We have showed a dramatic up regulation of RUNX2 expression with concomitant up-regulation of EGFR, IGF-1R and AXL, in melanoma cells rendered resistant to BRAF mutant inhibitors. Approximately half of melanomas carry BRAF mutations which enhance tumor invasion and metastasis. In this chapter, we describe the potential mechanisms, leading to the upregulation of RUNX2 in melanoma with BRAF mutations. We also highlight the critical role of PI3K/AKT in the expression and activation of RUNX2, and its consequences on the regulation of many critical factors, controlling cancer invasion and metastasis.

Keywords: Cancer and metastasis, melanoma, RUNX2, BRAF, PI3K/AKT, Wnt, Pthlh and DLX5, EGFR, IGF-1R and AXL

1. Introduction

Runt-related transcription factor 2 (Runx2) belongs to RUNX family, consisting of three members, Runx1, Runx2, and Runx3. All members are highly conserved with a 128 amino acid DNA binding/protein binding domain runt. In contrast to other RUNX members, RUNX2 holds a variable poly-glutamine, poly-alanine repeat domain [1]. Natural discrepancy within this repeat could alter the transactivation potential of RUNX2 which acts as an evolutionary 'tuning button' for the control of suggested to skull shape. The role of Runx2 is critical in skeletal development, and its alteration or low expression often lead to skeletal dysplasia. Runx2 plays important role in the process of mesenchymal stem cells differentiation into osteoblasts, and ultimately to osteocyte. Runx2 is required for the proliferation of pre-osteoblasts in whole skeletons and mesenchymal cells in sutures. Indeed, Runx2 is required for the commitment of mesenchymal cells to osteoblast lineage cells [2]. Thus, Runx2 makes a condensed cell layer of uncommitted mesenchymal cells or osteoblast progenitors by increasing their proliferation and facilitates their differentiation into osteoblast

IntechOpen

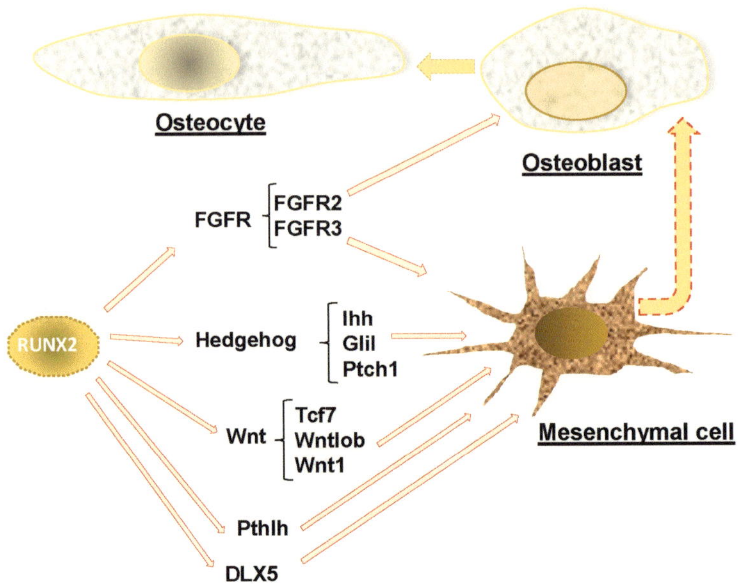

Figure 1.
RUNX2 and skeletal development. RUNX2 promotes osteoblast differentiation via several signaling pathways. RUNX2 directly acts on osteoblasts via Fgfr1 and Fgr2 to induce their differentiation and their promotion to osteocytes. RUNX2 acts on mesenchymal cells and induces specific pathways to enable osteoblast differentiation.

lineage cells. RUNX2 modulates the balance between osteoblasts and osteocytes, by either stimulating or inhibiting the osteoblast differentiation, occurring via the modulation of many factors and signaling pathways, including hedgehog signaling (Gli1, Ptch1 and Ihh), FGFR signaling (FGFR2 and FGFR3), Wnt signaling (Tcf7 and Wnt10b), Pth1r, Dlx5, Tnc, and Ncam1 (**Figure 1**). Defects or alterations in the expression or the activity of these factors or signaling pathways, may lead to skeletal dysplasia. Therefore, Runx2 could be used as target for the development of novel therapeutic strategies for bone-related diseases.

Besides, it is critical role in osteoblast differentiation, RUNX2 is also involved in the regulation of chondrocyte proliferation during bone formation. However, Runx2 expression in terminal hypertrophic chondrocytes is not essential for vascular invasion into the cartilage, but is for their survival and trans-differentiation into osteoblasts. Studies in animal models, showed that the trans-differentiation is required for trabecular bone formation in embryonic and neonatal stages, but not for procuring normal bone structure and volume in young and elder animals [3].

2. Multifaceted role of RUNX2 in cancer

The role of RUNX2 in cancer promotion has been well described in many cancer types. The common feature of those cancers is the elevated level of RUNX2 expression. Although, numerous similarities have been reported for the pro oncogenic role of RUNX2, some differences are also described (**Figure 2**).

In breast cancer (BC), early studies have shown a correlation between RUNX2 expression and the "Triple Negative" phenotype [4]. Analysis of tissue microarrays shown that high level of RUNX2 expression is associated with the triple-negative breast cancer phenotype and a low survival of BC patients, in comparison with patients, displaying reduced level of RUNX2 expression. Apparently, in triple negative cells, RUNX2 promotes Wnt and TGF-beta signaling [5]. RUNX2 is capable

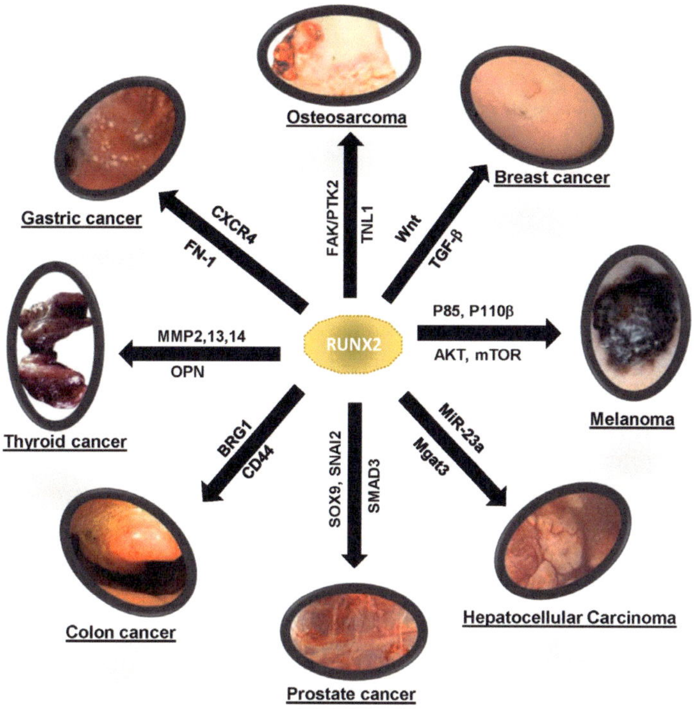

Figure 2.
RUNX2 and promotion of cancer. RUNX2 promotes cancer development of several cancer types: Melanoma, hepatocellular carcinoma, prostate cancer, colon cancer, thyroid cancer, gastric cancer, osteosarcoma and breast cancer. To promote cancer progression, RUNX2 induces several pathways, relevant to each cancer type.

to regulate different factors, playing critical role in either inhibiting or stimulating Wnt pathway. RUNX2 can interact with SMAD3 to promote TGF-beta signaling, in addition, to its direct interaction with the Estrogen receptor-alpha (ER-α), enabling the expression of aromatase, an estrogen producing enzyme. Increasing the level of estrogens, which in turn stimulate cell proliferation of BC cells [5].

It has been also reported that RUNX2 directly regulates TGFβ-induced levels of PTHrP, the level of MMP13 and MMP9, IL-8, bone sialoprotein and OPN [6–11]. Furthermore, we and others found that irregularities in RUNX2 expression induce EMT changes in some mammary epithelial cell lines and twists normal acini structure [6, 11, 12], strongly suggesting that RUNX2 plays a critical role in early breast cancer progression [6].

More recently, it has been demonstrated that RUNX2 was involved in breast cancer bone metastasis. This pro-metastatic role is mediated through integrin alpha5 [13].

In hepatocellular carcinoma (HCC), a significant increase of RUNX2 has been established in both HCC samples and cell lines. It has been demonstrated that RUNX2 promotes HCC cell migration and invasion via MMP9 [14]. In addition, RUNX2 increases the pro-metastatic process via MiR-23a and Mgat3 direct targeting [15].

In prostate cancer, RUNX2 has been also reported as cancer promotor. When RUNX2 is overexpressed in a C4-2B prostate cancer cell line, the invasiveness is greatly enhanced, and transcription factors involved in EMT (SOX9, SNAI2, and SMAD3) are upregulated [6, 16]. RUNX2 siRNA treatment of the prostate and breast cancer cells decreased migration and invasion of the cancerous cells [6, 17].

In gastric cancer (GC), a correlation between RUNX2 expression and invasion/metastasis has been established. Patients with GC tumors displaying low RUNX2 expression had a better outcome than those with high RUNX2 expression [18, 19]. RUNX2 was identified as an independent prognostic indicator for GC patients with a COX regression analysis. In an orthopedic GC nude mouse model, RUNX2 significantly increased the invasion and metastatic potential of the GC cells. *In vitro* studies reflected a significant increase in migration and invasion abilities of GC cells connected to an increase in RUNX2.

RUNX2 promotes metastasis and invasiveness of GC cells, via the chemokine receptor CXCR4 [18]. RUNX2 directly binds to the promotor region of CXCR4, enhancing its transcription and leading to overexpression in human GC cells. Knockdown of RUNX2 in GC cell lines results in a significant downregulation of CXCR4 mRNA. Additionally, CXCR4 is found to have a role in early-stage GC development by recruiting stromal cells and establishing a progenitor niche that favors tumor growth and development. However, it has been recently demonstrated that RUNX2 can negatively regulate the expression of Febronectin1 (FN1) [19], an important gene, playing critical role in tumor invasiveness and metastasis of GC [20, 21].

The role of RUNX2 has been also described in colon cancer. It has been found that RUNX2 promoted cell proliferation and invasion of colon cancer cells via estrogen/ERbeta pathway [10]. More recently, it has been demonstrated that RUNX2 could interact with BRG1 to target CD44 for promoting invasion and migration of colorectal cancer cells [22]. It has been also recently reported that Integrative multi-omics analysis of a colon cancer cells with heterogeneous Wnt activity reveals RUNX2 as an epigenetic regulator of Epithelial–mesenchymal transition (EMT), the critical process which promotes cancer metastasis, stemness and resistance to treatment [23].

The contribution of RUNX2 to the promotion of other cancer types, including thyroid cancer, osteosarcoma and melanoma has been also reported. RUNX2 activates expression of MMP2, MMP13, MMP14, and OPN, promoting the invasive and migratory activity of thyroid cancer cells [6, 24]. Osteosarcoma cells with siRNA depletion of RUNX2 show a reduction in motility. The genomic promoter of RUNX2 in osteosarcoma shows genes involved in cancer cell motility including FAK/PTK2 and TNL1 [6, 25]. The role of RUNx2 has been well studied in melanoma. Our group has extensively contributed to the understanding of the role of RUNX2 in this leading skin cancer.

3. Role of RUNX2 in melanoma promotion

Melanoma malignancy has a very high mortality rate and a resistance to chemotherapy [26]. Of these melanoma malignancies, a study reflected almost half of patients had bone metastases [27]. Melanocytes arise from the neural crest and show progressive stemness features. This renders melanoma to be such a highly metastatic cancer once the process has started [13]. Malignant melanoma has been described to have a higher expression level of RUNX2 than normal melanocytes [26]. As other cancer types, Runx2 has been investigated in connection to the progression, development, and metastasis of tumors as well as the epithelial to mesenchymal transition (EMT). It has been shown that the RUNT domain of RUNX2 affects EMT and promote bone metastasis in melanoma via several mechanisms, including WWTR1 and TGF-beta [26, 27].

The interaction of RUNX2 with the PI3K/AKT signaling pathway is critical for tumor invasion and metastasis [28]. AKT interacts with RUNX2 via different

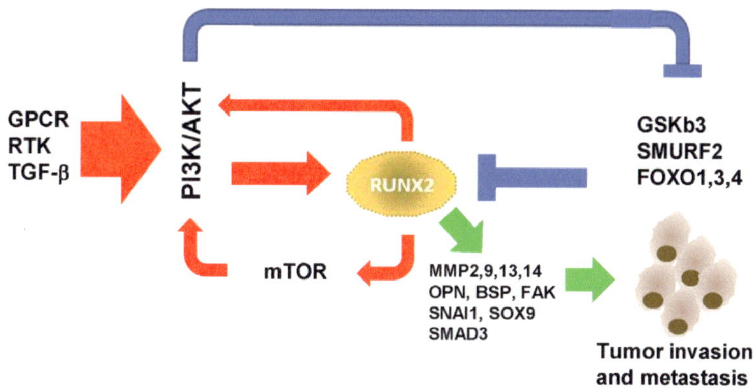

Figure 3.
Role RUNX2/PIT3K/AKT axis in cancer invasion and metastasis. PIT3/AKT promotes cancer invasion and metastasis via RUNX2. Activation loop between RUNX2 and PIT3/AKT enables the amplification of oncogenic signaling via many factors. Activation of RUNX2 lead to the promotion of cancer invasion and metastasis via the induction of MMPs and other factors.

mechanisms, including phosphorylating/activating of RUNX2 or RUNX2 modulators. Reciprocally, the activation of the PI3K/AKT pathway by RUNX2 has been also reported. This mutual activation, maintain a constitutive AKT activation and high expression of RUNX2 in cancer cells, and constitute one of a major driving force for tumor progression and metastasis in melanoma (**Figure 3**).

4. Role of RUNX2 in melanoma progression and acquired resistance to BRAFi

RUNX2 was initially described as one of the transcription factors whose expression was significantly correlated with elevated levels of the non-canonical signaling member of the WNT family, WNT5A, following chronic treatment (over 10 weeks) with the BRAF inhibitors PLX4720 and PLX4032 [29]. We previously showed that RUNX2-deficient melanoma cells, displayed a significant down-regulation of leading receptor tyrosine kinases, EGFR, IGF-1R, PDGFRβ and AXL. Our finding strongly suggested a critical role for RUNX2 in mediating intrinsic RTK-associated pro-oncogenic properties in melanoma. In addition, we demonstrated a significant up-regulation of RUNX2 expression and concomitant up-regulation of EGFR, IGF-1R and AXL in melanoma cells rendered resistant to PLX4720 [30]. We then reported that PLX4720-resistant cells developed in an *in vivo* context exhibit an increase in RUNX2 levels when re-exposed to PLX4720 *in vitro*. These findings strongly suggest that RUNX2 could play a critical role in acquired resistance to PLX4720. In order to address the relevance of these findings in human melanoma, clinical data from a cohort containing samples from untreated tumors and tumors treated with vemurafenib and dabrafenib respectively [31] were analyzed. Probes for all three main RUNX2 transcripts were represented on the array. We found that the expression of RUNX2 isoform 3 is significantly higher in vemurafenib-treated patients compared to the untreated group ($p = 0.0024$). These results showing the up-regulation of RUNX2 in melanoma lesions from patients treated with vemurafenib, strongly suggest that chronic exposure to BRAFi (PLX4720/vemurafenib) could favor RUNX2 up-regulation, leading to RTK up-regulation and the induction of acquired drug resistance to BRAFi [30].

The mechanism(s) leading to RUNX2 up-regulation in BRAFi-resistant melanoma cells have yet to be discovered. One possible mechanism would involve

WNT5A and the WNT5A-mediated activation of the PI3K/AKT pathway [29]. As RUNX2 expression is increased by the PI3K/AKT pathway signaling [28, 30], elevated WNT5A expression and subsequent AKT pathway activation could result in RUNX2 overexpression. Therefore, any kinase rewiring that leads to hyper-activated PI3K/AKT signaling in melanomas resistant to BRAFi [32] would provide a favorable context for high RUNX2 expression.

5. Conclusion

Besides, its indispensable role in bone development, the transcription factor RUNX2 is a critical player in the promotion of several cancers. Important oncogenic pathways, including PI3K/AKT axis are involved in mediating the effects of RUNX2. We believe that targeting RUNX2 or its modulators may open novel therapeutic avenues for cancer.

Acknowledgements

The authors thank all present and past laboratory members for their great contributions in progressing our understanding of RUNX2. American Cancer Society and NIH for funding.

Author details

Rachael Pulica[1], Karine Cohen Solal[1] and Ahmed Lasfar[1,2]*

1 Department of Pharmacology and Toxicology, Ernest Mario School of Pharmacy, Rutgers, The State University of New Jersey, Piscataway, NJ, United States

2 Rutgers-Cancer Institute of New Jersey, Rutgers University, New Brunswick, NJ, United States

*Address all correspondence to: lasfarah@gmail.com

References

[1] Newton, A.H. and Pask, A.J. (2020) Evolution and expansion of the RUNX2 QA repeat corresponds with the emergence of vertebrate complexity. Commun Biol, **3**, 771.

[2] Pokrovskaya, L.A., Nadezhdin, S.V., Zubareva, E.V., Burda, Y.E. and Gnezdyukova, E.S. (2020) Expression of RUNX2 and Osterix in Rat Mesenchymal Stem Cells during Culturing in Osteogenic-Conditioned Medium. Bull Exp Biol Med, **169**, 571-575.

[3] Qin, X., Jiang, Q., Nagano, K., Moriishi, T., Miyazaki, T., Komori, H., Ito, K., Mark, K.V., Sakane, C., Kaneko, H. *et al.* (2020) Runx2 is essential for the transdifferentiation of chondrocytes into osteoblasts. PLoS Genet, **16**, e1009169.

[4] Ferrari, N., McDonald, L., Morris, J.S., Cameron, E.R. and Blyth, K. (2013) RUNX2 in mammary gland development and breast cancer. J Cell Physiol, **228**, 1137-1142.

[5] Wysokinski, D., Blasiak, J. and Pawlowska, E. (2015) Role of RUNX2 in Breast Carcinogenesis. Int J Mol Sci, **16**, 20969-20993.

[6] Blyth, K., Vaillant, F., Jenkins, A., McDonald, L., Pringle, M.A., Huser, C., Stein, T., Neil, J. and Cameron, E.R. (2010) Runx2 in normal tissues and cancer cells: A developing story. Blood Cells Mol Dis, **45**, 117-123.

[7] Owens, T.W., Rogers, R.L., Best, S.A., Ledger, A., Mooney, A.M., Ferguson, A., Shore, P., Swarbrick, A., Ormandy, C.J., Simpson, P.T. *et al.* (2014) Runx2 is a novel regulator of mammary epithelial cell fate in development and breast cancer. Cancer Res, **74**, 5277-5286.

[8] Pratap, J., Imbalzano, K.M., Underwood, J.M., Cohet, N., Gokul, K., Akech, J., van Wijnen, A.J., Stein, J.L., Imbalzano, A.N., Nickerson, J.A. *et al.* (2009) Ectopic runx2 expression in mammary epithelial cells disrupts formation of normal acini structure: implications for breast cancer progression. Cancer Res, **69**, 6807-6814.

[9] Sancisi, V., Borettini, G., Maramotti, S., Ragazzi, M., Tamagnini, I., Nicoli, D., Piana, S. and Ciarrocchi, A. (2012) Runx2 isoform I controls a panel of proinvasive genes driving aggressiveness of papillary thyroid carcinomas. J Clin Endocrinol Metab, **97**, E2006-E2015.

[10] Sase, T., Suzuki, T., Miura, K., Shiiba, K., Sato, I., Nakamura, Y., Takagi, K., Onodera, Y., Miki, Y., Watanabe, M. *et al.* (2012) Runt-related transcription factor 2 in human colon carcinoma: a potent prognostic factor associated with estrogen receptor. Int J Cancer, **131**, 2284-2293.

[11] van der Deen, M., Akech, J., Lapointe, D., Gupta, S., Young, D.W., Montecino, M.A., Galindo, M., Lian, J.B., Stein, J.L., Stein, G.S. *et al.* (2012) Genomic promoter occupancy of runt-related transcription factor RUNX2 in Osteosarcoma cells identifies genes involved in cell adhesion and motility. J Biol Chem, **287**, 4503-4517.

[12] Boregowda, R.K., Olabisi, O.O., Abushahba, W., Jeong, B.S., Haenssen, K.K., Chen, W., Chekmareva, M., Lasfar, A., Foran, D.J., Goydos, J.S. *et al.* (2014) RUNX2 is overexpressed in melanoma cells and mediates their migration and invasion. Cancer Lett, **348**, 61-70.

[13] Li, X.Q., Lu, J.T., Tan, C.C., Wang, Q.S. and Feng, Y.M. (2016) RUNX2 promotes breast cancer bone metastasis by increasing integrin alpha5-mediated colonization. Cancer Lett, **380**, 78-86.

[14] Wang, Q., Yu, W., Huang, T., Zhu, Y. and Huang, C. (2016) RUNX2 promotes

hepatocellular carcinoma cell migration and invasion by upregulating MMP9 expression. Oncol Rep, **36**, 2777-2784.

[15] Huang, H., Liu, Y., Yu, P., Qu, J., Guo, Y., Li, W., Wang, S. and Zhang, J. (2018) MiR-23a transcriptional activated by Runx2 increases metastatic potential of mouse hepatoma cell via directly targeting Mgat3. Sci Rep, **8**, 7366.

[16] Pratap, J., Javed, A., Languino, L.R., van Wijnen, A.J., Stein, J.L., Stein, G.S. and Lian, J.B. (2005) The Runx2 osteogenic transcription factor regulates matrix metalloproteinase 9 in bone metastatic cancer cells and controls cell invasion. Mol Cell Biol, **25**, 8581-8591.

[17] Selvamurugan, N., Kwok, S. and Partridge, N.C. (2004) Smad3 interacts with JunB and Cbfa1/Runx2 for transforming growth factor-beta1-stimulated collagenase-3 expression in human breast cancer cells. J Biol Chem, **279**, 27764-27773.

[18] Guo, Z.J., Yang, L., Qian, F., Wang, Y.X., Yu, X., Ji, C.D., Cui, W., Xiang, D.F., Zhang, X., Zhang, P. *et al.* (2016) Transcription factor RUNX2 up-regulates chemokine receptor CXCR4 to promote invasive and metastatic potentials of human gastric cancer. Oncotarget, 7, 20999-21012.

[19] Han, C., Jin, L., Ma, X., Hao, Q., Lin, H. and Zhang, Z. (2020) Identification of the hub genes RUNX2 and FN1 in gastric cancer. Open Med (Wars), **15**, 403-412.

[20] Wang, J., Deng, L., Huang, J., Cai, R., Zhu, X., Liu, F., Wang, Q., Zhang, J. and Zheng, Y. (2017) High expression of Fibronectin 1 suppresses apoptosis through the NF-kappaB pathway and is associated with migration in nasopharyngeal carcinoma. Am J Transl Res, **9**, 4502-4511.

[21] Xu, X., Liu, Z., Zhou, L., Xie, H., Cheng, J., Ling, Q., Wang, J., Guo, H., Wei, X. and Zheng, S. (2015) Characterization of genome-wide TFCP2 targets in hepatocellular carcinoma: implication of targets FN1 and TJP1 in metastasis. J Exp Clin Cancer Res, **34**, 6.

[22] Yan, X., Han, D., Chen, Z., Han, C., Dong, W., Han, L., Zou, L., Zhang, J., Liu, Y. and Chai, J. (2020) RUNX2 interacts with BRG1 to target CD44 for promoting invasion and migration of colorectal cancer cells. Cancer Cell Int, **20**, 505.

[23] Yi, H., Li, G., Long, Y., Liang, W., Cui, H., Zhang, B., Tan, Y., Li, Y., Shen, L., Deng, D. *et al.* (2020) Integrative multi-omics analysis of a colon cancer cell line with heterogeneous Wnt activity revealed RUNX2 as an epigenetic regulator of EMT. Oncogene, **39**, 5152-5164.

[24] Sun, L., Vitolo, M. and Passaniti, A. (2001) Runt-related gene 2 in endothelial cells: inducible expression and specific regulation of cell migration and invasion. Cancer Res, **61**, 4994-5001.

[25] Kwon, T.G., Zhao, X., Yang, Q., Li, Y., Ge, C., Zhao, G. and Franceschi, R.T. (2011) Physical and functional interactions between Runx2 and HIF-1alpha induce vascular endothelial growth factor gene expression. J Cell Biochem, **112**, 3582-3593.

[26] Pratap, J., Lian, J.B. and Stein, G.S. (2011) Metastatic bone disease: role of transcription factors and future targets. Bone, **48**, 30-36.

[27] Sun, S.S., Zhang, L., Yang, J. and Zhou, X. (2015) Role of runt-related transcription factor 2 in signal network of tumors as an inter-mediator. Cancer Lett, **361**, 1-7.

[28] Cohen-Solal, K.A., Boregowda, R.K. and Lasfar, A. (2015) RUNX2 and the PI3K/AKT axis reciprocal activation as a

driving force for tumor progression. Mol Cancer, **14**, 137.

[29] Anastas, J.N., Kulikauskas, R.M., Tamir, T., Rizos, H., Long, G.V., von Euw, E.M., Yang, P.T., Chen, H.W., Haydu, L., Toroni, R.A. *et al.* (2014) WNT5A enhances resistance of melanoma cells to targeted BRAF inhibitors. J Clin Invest, **124**, 2877-2890.

[30] Boregowda, R.K., Medina, D.J., Markert, E., Bryan, M.A., Chen, W., Chen, S., Rabkin, A., Vido, M.J., Gunderson, S.I., Chekmareva, M. *et al.* (2016) The transcription factor RUNX2 regulates receptor tyrosine kinase expression in melanoma. Oncotarget, **7**, 29689-29707.

[31] Rizos, H., Menzies, A.M., Pupo, G.M., Carlino, M.S., Fung, C., Hyman, J., Haydu, L.E., Mijatov, B., Becker, T.M., Boyd, S.C. *et al.* (2014) BRAF inhibitor resistance mechanisms in metastatic melanoma: spectrum and clinical impact. Clin Cancer Res, **20**, 1965-1977.

[32] Paraiso, K.H., Xiang, Y., Rebecca, V.W., Abel, E.V., Chen, Y.A., Munko, A.C., Wood, E., Fedorenko, I.V., Sondak, V.K., Anderson, A.R. *et al.* (2011) PTEN loss confers BRAF inhibitor resistance to melanoma cells through the suppression of BIM expression. Cancer Res, **71**, 2750-2760.